# MY CHILD HAS CANCER

# MY CHILD HAS CANCER

## A Parent's Guide to Diagnosis, Treatment, and Survival

Della L. Howell, M.D.

The Praeger Series on Healing and Managing Injury and Disease
Julie K. Silver, M.D., Series Editor

PRAEGER

Westport, Connecticut
London

**Library of Congress Cataloging-in-Publication Data**

Howell, Della L., 1973–
    My child has cancer : a parent's guide to diagnosis, treatment, and survival /
    Della L. Howell.
        p. cm. — (Praeger series on healing and managing injury and disease,
        ISSN 1940–5804)
    Includes bibliographical references and index.
    ISBN 978–0–275–99601–7 (alk. paper)
1. Cancer in children—Popular works. I. Title.
RC281.C4H69 2008
618.92′994—dc22        2007048298

British Library Cataloguing in Publication Data is available.

Library of Congress Catalog Card Number: 2007048298
ISBN: 978–0–275–99601–7
ISSN: 1940–5804

First published in 2008

Praeger Publishers, 88 Post Road West, Westport, CT 06881
An imprint of Greenwood Publishing Group, Inc.
www.praeger.com

Printed in the United States of America

The paper used in this book complies with the
Permanent Paper Standard issued by the National
Information Standards Organization (Z39.48–1984).

10 9 8 7 6 5 4 3 2 1

For Clay, Will, Emily Grace, and Rachel

# CONTENTS

# SERIES FOREWORD

Pediatric hematologist/oncologist Della Howell writes in the opening pages of this book about one of her favorite words—*children*—and one of her most dreaded—*cancer*. Combining these two words is the subject matter for her professional life and the content of this wonderful guide for families.

Ideally, one would never use *children* and *cancer* in the same sentence, but in fact the incidence of pediatric cancer is increasing (though survival rates are too, fortunately). Serious illness is not just reserved for adults—kids can get cancer, and when they do, their families face the overwhelming task of getting the information they need to successfully navigate the health care system, seek out appropriate treatment, and help their child physically and emotionally recover as well as possible.

Where to begin? Dr. Howell has written just the guide in *My Child Has Cancer: A Parent's Guide to Diagnosis, Treatment, and Survival.*

In a thoughtful, thorough, and highly readable book, Dr. Howell guides readers through the diagnosis and treatment phases and offers strategies to help them cope. Between the lines, readers will find a sincere and empathic woman who is an expert in both the science of pediatric oncology and the support that families need to face this difficult journey.

Dr. Howell is a mother, wife, physician, and accomplished pianist. She has much to offer the families of children diagnosed with cancer in this important book. The future for pediatric oncology looks brighter and brighter,

but the journey is still long and very difficult. In this guide, Dr. Howell helps
to pave the way.

Julie K. Silver, M.D.
Series Editor

# INTRODUCTION

*A four-year-old girl sits on a hospital gurney in the emergency room. She seems scared and a little overwhelmed by all of the lights and noises of the hospital. Her dark brown eyes have a sense of sadness as she sits there, very still and quiet. She stares at the floor, rarely looking at my face. The girl's mother is there with her, standing beside the gurney, stroking her daughter's curly brown hair, keeping strands away from her face.*

*As I close the curtain, the mother's attention turns towards me with a look of mild concern. I start to ask questions: How long has the girl been sick? Why did she come to the emergency room? Has she been healthy in the past? What are her symptoms? The mother tells me that Sara is there because she was having knee pain and fevers. She has never been sick before. The emergency room doctors told the mother that there was a problem with Sara's blood tests. Unfortunately, I already know that there is a problem—that's why I am seeing Sara.*

*I am a pediatric oncologist, so I specialize in taking care of children and adolescents with cancer. I received a phone call only minutes before, telling me that a young girl's lab tests showed leukemia. I already know some of the child's symptoms and health background, but I need to talk to Sara's mother before breaking the life-shattering news that her daughter has cancer.*

*We start talking about the blood test and the specific things that the other doctors noted. Then I tell her that I am very concerned that her beautiful young daughter has leukemia. She starts sobbing uncontrollably. I have no idea what to do—should I keep talking? Should I get someone else for the mother? Should I just leave? It is so hard to know that you are responsible for giving such horrendous, unbelievable news to a family that, up until now, has been "normal."*

*After she has a chance to compose herself and spend time with Sara, I try to prepare them for what will happen next. More blood tests. Hospital stays. Procedures. Medications. I'm not sure that she has heard a word that I've said, but I had to start somewhere. I try to talk to her in a manner that I would want to be addressed. I always try to put myself in the minds of the people that I'm speaking to, staying empathetic, considerate, never rushing. They deserve to have the undivided attention and compassion of the person who can help make the cancer go away. As far as I am concerned at this moment, Sara is the* only *patient in the world. Sara and her mother deserve nothing less than my best.*

*Children.* This is one of my favorite words. I think of children and I can't help but smile. Their innocence, their carefree nature, the way that they say whatever comes to their minds—these are all wonderful things in a world that, at times, seems filled with trouble.

*Cancer.* This is one of the most dreaded words I know. It strikes fear in most peoples' hearts. Yet, almost everyone has been affected at some time in life by cancer, whether through a parent, a friend, or their own personal experiences.

In an ideal world, the words *children* and *cancer* would never share a sentence. Unfortunately, children can and do get cancer, and when this happens, a family's world is shattered. How could someone so innocent get such a devastating disease? When a child is given this diagnosis, the family bears the burden for the rest of their lives. It affects not only the child's physical health, but the emotional health of the child, parents, siblings, extended family members, friends, classmates, and teachers. It places a strain on relationships both within the family and outside the family.

The family of a child with cancer very quickly forms a relationship with the medical community—doctors, nurses, hospitals, clinics, and pharmacies. This relationship should be a strong one, one that can be a source of support for the family and the child during one of the most difficult times in their lives. I truly love being a part of that community, working closely with these children and their families, helping them through some unbelievably difficult moments.

People often ask how I can do this job—how I can treat and take care of children with cancer. "It must be so depressing." "I couldn't bear to see all those sick children." "How are you able to sleep at night?" I always tell them that I am privileged to take care of some of the best patients and families possible, and I couldn't imagine working anywhere else. These patients are *my* patients. The children, their families, and the hospital staff work together to get the children through one of the worst times in their lives. In many instances, I don't just feel like their physician; I feel like a member of their family. We all have the same goal—a cure.

In 1998, in the United States there were 12,400 children and adolescents younger than 20 years of age diagnosed with cancer. Almost 2,500 children and adolescents died of cancer during this same year. The incidence of pediatric cancer has increased significantly since the mid-1970s. However, thanks to wonderful advances in modern medicine, the survival rates have also improved during this time. Despite the improvement in survival as a whole, cancer is still the most common cause of disease-related mortality in these age groups, so even more work is needed to come up with the ideal cure for all types of cancer.

But until that cure is discovered, families hunger for information when a loved one is diagnosed with cancer. It is a frightening disease that can be devastating. I know this not just as a doctor, but as a cancer patient. I was diagnosed with metastatic carcinoid cancer of the small intestine in late 2006, just a month before the youngest daughter of my three children turned one. Hearing that I had a type of cancer with no truly effective treatment was very difficult to handle, but I actually received strength when I thought of my patients and their struggles. These children face tremendous obstacles in their fight against cancer. If they could take on the war, so could I.

While there are many resources available, the information can be fragmented, complicated, or not detailed enough for family members. In this book, I attempt to provide accurate, in-depth information for parents and other family members of children or teenagers with cancer. The book is also meant as a resource for those who just want to learn more about the journey that begins when a child or young adult is found to have cancer. In the book, I cover areas such as the differences between cancer in children and cancer in adults; treatment of cancer, including chemotherapy, bone marrow transplant, and "alternative" therapies; and coping with some of the future struggles met by children who have completed therapy for cancer.

I am honored to work in this field of medicine. I have been given the opportunity to work with some of the most compassionate healthcare workers, strongest families, and sweetest children in the world. While we don't always win our battles with cancer, I leave work every day believing that I have been able to make a real difference in the life of a child and in the lives of their family members.

It is my hope that this book will bring you information and understanding. And with this understanding, each reader will find strength.

# ABBREVIATIONS

| | |
|---|---|
| 6-MP | mercaptopurine |
| 6-TG | thioguanine |
| AFP | alpha-fetoprotein |
| ALCL | anaplastic large cell lymphoma |
| ALL | acute lymphoblastic leukemia |
| AML | acute myelogenous leukemia |
| ANC | absolute neutrophil count |
| ARA-C | cytarabine |
| B-HCG | beta-human chorionic gonadotropin |
| BMT | bone marrow transplant |
| CAHCIM | Consortium of Academic Health Centers for Integrative Medicine |
| CAM | complementary and alternative medicine |
| CBC | complete blood count |
| CML | chronic myelogenous leukemia |
| CNS | central nervous system |
| COG | Children's Oncology Group |
| CSF | cerebrospinal fluid |
| CT | computed tomography |
| DMSO | dimethyl sulfoxide |
| DNA | deoxyribonucleic acid |
| DO | doctor of osteopathy |
| EBV | Epstein Barr Virus |
| ECG/EKG | electrocardiogram |
| ER | Emergency Room |
| ESR | erythrocyte sedimentation rate |
| FAB | French-American-British |

| FDA | Food and Drug Administration |
| FNA | fine needle aspiration |
| GBM | glioblastoma multiforme |
| GVHD | graft versus host disease |
| HCC | hepatocellular carcinoma |
| HIV | Human Immunodeficiency Virus |
| HLA | human leukocyte antigen |
| HVA | homovanillic acid |
| IM | integrative medicine |
| IRB | Institutional Review Board |
| IV | intravenous |
| JPA | juvenile pilocytic astrocytoma |
| LDH | lactate dehydrogenase |
| LVN | licensed vocational nurse |
| MD | medical doctor |
| MDS | myelodysplastic syndrome |
| MIBG | metaiodobenzylguanidine |
| MRI | magnetic resonance imaging |
| NCCAM | National Center for Complementary and Alternative Medicine |
| NCI | National Cancer Institute |
| NHL | non-Hodgkin lymphoma |
| NIH | National Institutes of Health |
| NRSTS | non-rhabdomyosarcoma soft tissue sarcoma |
| PACU | post-anesthesia care unit |
| PET | positron emission tomography |
| PFT | pulmonary function test |
| PICC | peripherally inserted central catheter |
| PICU | Pediatric intensive care unit |
| PNET | primitive neuroectodermal tumor |
| RN | registered nurse |
| SCT | stem cell transplant |
| TBI | total body irradiation |
| TPN | total parenteral nutrition |
| VMA | vanillylmandelic acid |
| VOD | veno-occlusive disease |
| WBC | white blood cell |
| WHO | World Health Organization |

# Chapter 1

## CANCER AND CHILDREN

### WHAT IS CANCER?

Simply put, cancer is an abnormal growth of cells. Cells are the building blocks for our body; there are many different kinds of cells within our bodies, and the type of cancer depends on the type of cell from which it started. For example, leukemia (cancer of the blood) usually comes from white blood cells, while sarcomas (a type of solid tumor) originate from muscle cells. The name of each type of cancer gives you a clue about where the cancer is located and which type of cell is responsible for its growth.

Cancer cells develop because of a change in a normal cell's DNA (deoxyribonucleic acid). DNA is essentially a genetic code for an individual. It helps determine the individual characteristics for each person. The normal cells in a person's body divide rapidly and duplicate the DNA in a very intricate process. Billions of cells are dividing in our bodies on a daily basis, and errors will occur. Fortunately, the body has a built-in repair mechanism to fix these errors, so usually these mistakes don't cause problems in the body. The problems occur when the errors go unnoticed. An "abnormal" cancer cell gets through the natural checks and balances of the body and is allowed to divide and duplicate its own abnormal DNA, eventually leading to the disease of cancer. Cancer cells grow and divide more quickly than our body's normal cells, so the cancerous growth overtakes the normal growth, leading to symptoms.

## Why Does Cancer Happen?

What allows the error to happen? What truly causes cancer? There are several theories on the subject, but sadly, no one has all the answers. Scientists are fairly confident with the generalization that DNA is the source of the problem, but there are many potential reasons for abnormal DNA. Some believe that viruses are to blame for most cancers, but it's hard to accept that this is the whole answer. If a particular virus is the sole reason for a certain type of cancer developing, then why don't more of those in close contact with those who have cancer also develop cancer? Usually, when a virus hits a family with cold symptoms or gastrointestinal upset, many people who share close quarters become sick with the same type of infection. This is not the case with cancer.

## Genetics in Cancer

Others think that the genes we inherit are to blame, and in some cases, we know that this is true. People who have many relatives in their family with particular types of cancers, such as brain cancer, bone cancer, or breast cancer, are oftentimes more likely to get cancer themselves. However, this does not explain all incidences of cancer, because there are many people who develop cancer who have no family members with cancer. Our bodies have some genes that are considered "tumor suppressor" genes, and we may have others that are called "proto-oncogenes." Tumor suppressor genes do what their name says—they suppress the growth of tumors, or cancer. If these genes become defective, they can't do their job, and a person is more likely to develop cancer. Proto-oncogenes are genes that in basic terms actually lead to the formation of cancer ("proto" can be combined with other words to mean that word's ancestor; and "onco" is a word for cancer—think "oncologist"). If a person has inherited one of these proto-oncogenes from a parent, then he has inherited a "genetic ancestor for cancer." This leads to the belief that these people are therefore more likely to develop cancer than those who have a more normal genetic background.

## Cancer and the Environment

Another theory is that environmental exposures lead to the development of cancer. Smoking and radiation are two examples of environmental exposures that are associated with increased risks of cancer. However, of two separate individuals who have the same amount of cigarette exposure or radiation exposure, one might get cancer, while the other might not. What makes one person more likely to get cancer than the other? Unfortunately, there is no answer to this question, yet.

## Cancer Comes from a Combination of Factors

A more likely explanation is a multifactorial one, as was first presented by Dr. Alfred G. Knudson in the Knudson hypothesis—multiple "hits" on the body are required for a specific individual to get cancer. Perhaps a virus provides one "hit" on a person's body, making a subtle change in that person's DNA. Then, an environmental exposure such as smoking gives the second "hit," leading to another small change in that same person's DNA. And if that same person has bad genes (a brother with a brain tumor, an uncle with bone cancer, a mother with breast cancer), this is the final "hit" required to make this person develop cancer.

## Adults Versus Children with Cancer

When most people think of cancer, they may think of an older relative or friend who had breast cancer, lung cancer, colon cancer, or prostate cancer, which are four of the most common types of cancer in adults (Table 1.1). Adults are often not completely healthy when they get cancer; they may have

**Table 1.1   Estimated Yearly Incidence of Cancer in Adults and Pediatric (<20 years of age) Patients**

| Adults[1] | | Children/Adolescents[2] | |
|---|---|---|---|
| Type of cancer | Incidence | Type of cancer | Incidence |
| Skin (non-melanoma) | >1,000,000 | Leukemia | 3,250 |
| Prostate | 234,460 | Brain tumors | 2,200 |
| Breast | 214,640 | Lymphoma | 1,700 |
| Lung | 174,470 | Neuroblastoma | 650 |
| Colon and Rectal | 148,610 | Wilms' tumor | 500 |
| Melanoma | 62,190 | Osteosarcoma | 400 |
| Bladder | 61,420 | Rhabdomyosarcoma | 350 |
| Non-Hodgkins Lymphoma | 58,870 | Thyroid carcinoma | 350 |
| Endometrial | 41,200 | Melanoma | 300 |
| Leukemia (All) | 35,070 | Retinoblastoma | 300 |

*Sources:* 1) American Cancer Society: Cancer Facts and Figures 2006. Atlanta, GA: American Cancer Society, 2006. 2) Cancer Incidence and Survival among Children and Adolescents: United States SEER Program 1975–1995.

heart disease, diabetes, or other chronic medical problems that predispose them to having infectious complications, fatigue, or chronic pain. Adults are often unable to tolerate intense cancer treatment regimens because of poor baseline health.

Pediatric cancer is quite different from adult cancer. The most common types of cancer in children are leukemia, brain tumors, neuroblastoma, and Wilms' tumor (more details about these diseases will be covered in the next chapter). Children are usually in good health prior to presenting with cancer symptoms and only rarely have to deal with chronic medical problems during their cancer treatment. They can tolerate intense treatment regimens much better than their adult counterparts.

Another important difference between adult cancer and pediatric cancer is the concept of "survival." Somewhere between 70–80 percent of all pediatric cancer patients will become long-term survivors, with definite variability according to the type of cancer. Unfortunately, adults usually don't fare as well. However, when looking at terms like "five-year survival" from cancer, which is a major landmark for most adults dealing with cancer, this statistic is not as exciting for children.

Imagine a 70-year-old man who develops lung cancer and a 3-year-old girl who develops leukemia. Five years for the man with lung cancer gets him to a more acceptable length of life; five years for the young girl doesn't even get her to fourth grade. The focus on truly lengthening the life of children who are afflicted with cancer guides a lot of the therapies for pediatric cancer. Physicians are more aggressive in treatment and want to actually cure the patient of the disease so they can have a long and fruitful life. For adults, sometimes the best treatment is something that doesn't cause a lot of side effects but merely gives a good quality of life with a shorter extension of time.

# Chapter 2

# TYPES OF CANCER, PART I—LEUKEMIA

In these sections, the focus is on the individual types of cancer that commonly affect children. Details on the specific therapies used to fight cancer will be discussed in detail in a later chapter.

## LEUKEMIA

*My son James was always such a healthy boy—never sick, never absent from school. He had never seen a doctor except for routine "physical" visits. When he started running fevers, I thought that he just had a virus like most children. A couple of days later, he was still having fevers and seemed so tired. He didn't want to play. He didn't want to go outside. This was not my child. A family friend told me that she thought he looked "pale." He was also having nosebleeds and these little red dots on his skin. When I took him to the pediatrician, she recommended that we get some blood work on James. An hour after the blood was taken, she called us back into the office, sat us down, and said that James had leukemia. I didn't know what leukemia was. I just knew it was bad. I was even more shocked when the Pediatrician said that leukemia was cancer. My son can't have cancer, I thought. Cancer is for old people. Cancer kills people. My son can't die. People with cancer lose their hair and feel sick and are miserable. Over the next few days, James saw many different doctors and had many tests. Some were painful, some were simple. I came to learn more about leukemia, and I realized that this was something that James could and would beat! He is now 2 years into his treatment and overall doing well.*

*The beginning was the worst. Each day gets a little bit easier. Each day gets us a little bit closer to knowing that he can be cured of this disease. [Excerpt from a conversation with a mother of a child with leukemia.]*

Leukemia is the most common cancer in children. It is a cancer of the blood cells, so some people think of it as a "liquid" cancer. However, it can also be present in "solid" structures in the body, such as lymph nodes (described below), the liver, and the spleen. Leukemia is a very broad diagnosis. There are many different subtypes of this disease that affect children, and the specific subtype is important in deciding on the best treatment for the child and for the overall prognosis.

**The Bone Marrow and Blood Cells**

Before discussing the various types of leukemia, we need to understand a little bit about the blood cells in the body. Blood is made in the bone marrow; this is considered the "factory" for the body's blood cells. Most people can conceptualize bone marrow better if they think of a chicken or turkey bone. If this bone is broken, you will notice a dark discoloration in the middle of the bone; this is the bone marrow. It is actually a liquid substance that looks an awful lot like regular blood when you see it in a specimen container. The abnormal cancer cells in leukemia, also called "blasts," start being made in the bone marrow. Once the cancer has grown enough in the bone marrow, the cells usually start to be released into the blood stream, and the diagnosis of leukemia is easier at this stage.

There are three groups of blood cells in the body: red blood cells, platelets, and white blood cells. Red blood cells are the cells that carry oxygen throughout the body. If someone is "anemic," they have a problem with their red blood cells. If you look at a red blood cell under the microscope, it has the shape of a doughnut. Illnesses like sickle cell disease and iron-deficiency anemia are processes that involve the red blood cells.

Platelets are the smallest blood cells. They are involved in the clotting of the blood. When a person has a cut or scrape on the skin or a bruise under the skin, the platelets are part of the process of making the bleeding stop or keeping the bruise from spreading too much.

White blood cells are the cells that help us fight infection. There are several different types of white blood cells in any normal person. Neutrophils (otherwise known as granulocytes or segs) are typically thought of as cells that help with bacterial infections. Neutrophils are involved in the formation of pus. Lymphocytes are another type of white blood cell, and they have an important function in the body's immune system and memory of previous infections. Monocytes, eosinophils, and basophils are usually present in small numbers in most healthy individuals, and they may have some significance in certain kinds of infections or other illnesses. In the majority of people with leukemia, the white blood cells are the source of the disease.

When leukemia cells fill the bone marrow, there is no room left for the factory to produce "normal" cells. This leads to a lot of the symptoms of leukemia. Children may become anemic, which may cause them to be tired and pale. They may show signs of excessive bruising of the skin (bruises in strange places, abnormally large bruises) or unexpected bleeding (often of the gums). They may also develop tiny little red dots, called petechiae, on various parts of the body. This is because they are unable to make normal numbers of platelets. Children may also have significant infections that aren't responding to the usual antibiotic treatment because there are no normal white blood cells present to help fight infections. The degree of suppression of these normal cells varies from child to child, and this changes the symptoms of presentation as well.

### Acute Versus Chronic Leukemia

Leukemia has two basic types of presentation. There is acute leukemia, which is more common in children (comprising 98 percent of childhood leukemia cases) and has a more sudden onset, as its name describes. Chronic leukemia (the other 2 percent of childhood leukemia cases) is more common in adults than in children, and comes about more slowly. Each type can share some of the same symptoms at presentation, but other symptoms are more common in either acute or chronic forms of leukemia.

### Presenting Signs and Symptoms

Fever and fatigue are often present at the diagnosis of leukemia. Many parents say that their child has had fevers off and on for a couple of weeks, sometimes treated with antibiotics without a response. Some children have an infection that is causing the fever, but the infection is not responding to the usual treatments. Fatigue may have been going on for days to weeks in children, and this can be related to anemia, or prolonged infections.

Bone pain often occurs in children with leukemia because of the expansion of the bone marrow. This swelling of the fluid within the bone increases the pressure, leading to pain. This pain tends to be the greatest in the longer bones of the body, such as the legs. Children with acute leukemia may present with joint pain and swelling, or pallor (paleness to the skin and/or lips). They may have significant bruising or bleeding if their platelet counts are too low.

Sometimes children with acute leukemia will have enlarged lymph nodes. Lymph nodes are part of the body's lymphatic system. You can find lymph nodes in many areas of the body. The most common regions for enlarged lymph nodes in children are the neck, under the arms, and in the groin, but they can also be found deep inside the chest, abdomen, or pelvis, or even in areas behind the knees or around the elbows. They are involved in the immune system and its response to infections, so they are often enlarged in illnesses like strep throat or skin abscesses. Many children have lymph nodes that can be felt even at times when they are healthy, but these tend to be less than one to two centimeters (or about half an inch) in size. When they are enlarged in infections, they are usually somewhat tender, and in an area of the body close to a known infection. Picture a child with a sore throat who also has tender lumps in his neck. When they are enlarged in relation to leukemia, they may be rock-hard, non-tender, and in many different areas of the body.

Another symptom of leukemia is something called hepatosplenomegaly. This means that the liver and spleen are both enlarged. (You can also have just hepatomegaly—enlargement of the liver—or splenomegaly—enlargement of the spleen.) These organs, found in the upper abdomen, tend to become enlarged from leukemia cells that get trapped. The liver is located on the right, and the spleen is located on the left. Enlargement of these organs can lead to their own set of symptoms, such as abdominal pain or what looks like abdominal swelling.

In males, sometimes testicular enlargement is noted when they present with leukemia. Leukemia cells can actually infiltrate the testes and cause a mass within one or both of the testicles.

**Testing for Leukemia**

Doctors will perform many blood tests in children where the diagnosis of leukemia is suspected. The most important of these blood tests is the Complete Blood Count, or CBC. The CBC is a test that says whether or not the white blood cell counts, red blood cell counts, and platelets are normal or abnormal. In the majority of cases of leukemia, the child will present with abnormal numbers in some or all of these areas. The CBC is run through a machine, which analyzes the blood specimen very carefully. When the machine gets unexpected results, in most instances a laboratory technician will make a "smear" or microscope slide of the blood so that it can be double-checked by human eyes. These slides are often reviewed by the pathologists or oncologists if there are concerns for leukemia blasts being seen. This test can be performed fairly quickly in most centers, within a matter of minutes to a couple of hours.

It is important to know that not every child with leukemia will have these blasts in their blood stream, or peripheral blood, so a simple blood test cannot give the answer. Occasionally, the physician must obtain a sample of the bone marrow to make the diagnosis. The bone marrow can also be placed on a microscope slide for review by the pathologist or oncologist. This test typically takes a little longer and often requires more planning. More information on bone marrow testing will be given in a later chapter.

A more definitive test for leukemia is a laboratory test called flow cytometry. In this test, a specimen of blood or bone marrow is put through a machine that is able to separate and analyze the specific types of blood cells for certain markers or antigens that belong in particular types of leukemia. The normal blood cells are removed from the picture so the doctor can focus attention on the abnormal cells. The test can also say how much of the blood is abnormal in terms of percentages. Flow cytometry is the easiest and most accurate way at this time to give the specific subtype of leukemia, and results are usually available in a matter of hours.

After a diagnosis of leukemia is made, the doctors will want to see if the leukemia has spread to another area of the body—the spinal fluid. This examination requires a more invasive test, which is a spinal tap, otherwise known as a lumbar puncture. The spinal tap is done to obtain a sample of cerebrospinal fluid (CSF) (procedure discussed in more detail in a later chapter). Unfortunately, leukemia cells are smart—they know which places in the body give them a "safe haven." The brain or CSF is one of these places. There is something called the blood-brain-barrier, which is a barrier in place to help protect the brain from various outside toxins, such as medications. Leukemia cells that are able to infiltrate this area are naturally protected from some forms of medical treatment because of the brain's own defense system. Approximately 6–12 percent of children with leukemia will have leukemia cells noted in the spinal fluid at the time of diagnosis. This central nervous system, or CNS, leukemia can have symptoms of headaches, problems with balance, and vision changes associated with the disease in the spinal fluid.

**Progression of Leukemic Disease**

Obviously, the goal in treating leukemia is to cure the patient of the disease. However, the word "cure" is not used until a significant amount of time has passed since the time of diagnosis. For many, "cure" comes when a patient has gone five years with no signs that the cancer is coming back.

The more appropriate term to use during the initial treatments for leukemia is "remission." Remission occurs at the first time that there is no evidence of any disease. For leukemia patients, this means that the bone marrow contains less than 5 percent leukemia cells, or blast cells, with other cells being normal in number, and that there are no other signs or symptoms of disease.

Most patients are in remission following the first few weeks of treatment. When the leukemia doesn't go into remission at the appropriate time, oncologists worry that the leukemia is not as sensitive to the chemotherapy treatments. These patients often receive more aggressive therapy. There are rare instances of patients with leukemia who never achieve a state of remission. Unfortunately, remission must occur before a cure, and patients who do not experience remission usually die of their disease.

In recent years, special tests have been developed that are better at detecting leukemia cells. These tests can pick up even tiny amounts of leukemia blasts. When the blasts are still present, but in very small numbers, physicians refer to this as "minimal residual disease." Patients that have minimal residual disease are still technically "in remission," but they also seem to need more aggressive therapy to be eventually cured of their cancer.

### Acute Lymphoblastic Leukemia

Acute Lymphoblastic Leukemia (ALL) is the most common form of leukemia affecting children. It accounts for 78 percent of leukemia cases in children 15 years of age and younger, and 50 percent of leukemia cases in adolescents between the ages of 15 and 19 years.[1] As its name states, it is one of the types of leukemia that has an acute (sudden) onset. Children often present with fevers, fatigue, or bone or joint pain. The lymph nodes are often enlarged, and the liver or spleen might be enlarged as well. This is also the most common type of leukemia to affect the testicles.

ALL is most likely to present in children between the ages of two and eight, with a peak incidence around four years of age, but it can strike at any time of life from infancy to adulthood. It is more likely to affect males than females. Certain basic features can make children high-risk or low-risk in terms of how aggressive the leukemia will be. These features include age at diagnosis (higher risk for those less than one year of age or greater than ten years of age), total number of white blood cells noted on the CBC (higher risk for white blood cell count greater than 50,000/uL, which is five to ten times the normal range), and certain subtypes of leukemia cells within this group. Children who have leukemia in their spinal fluid at the time of their diagnosis are also considered to be in a high-risk group.

*Lymphoblast* is the specific name of the cell that is involved in this type of leukemia. In essence, a lymphoblast is a cancerous lymphocyte. When a lymphocyte develops in the bone marrow, it has to go through different stages of growth and maturation. One of the earliest stages of growth is that of a lymphoblast. Normally, lymphoblasts should all differentiate (grow up, become more mature) into the more mature lymphocyte. In ALL, the altered DNA of the cells causes the lymphoblasts to grow in numbers without differentiating or maturing into normal lymphocytes. These lymphoblasts are not really functional for the body, they are not as helpful in fighting infections, and their tremendous growth keeps the bone marrow from being able to make normal blood cells.

There are different types of lymphoblastic leukemia as well, with each name being a representation of the type of lymphocyte that is affected. Two of the major types of small lymphocytes are T- and B-lymphocytes. The most common subtype of lymphoblastic leukemia is precursor-B ALL (pre-B ALL). The lymphoblasts in this situation are early or precursor-B lymphoblasts, and they have a very specific "fingerprint" found on the flow cytometry testing described above. There are also leukemias referred to as T-cell ALL and B-cell ALL (also known as Burkitt's leukemia). Knowing the specific subtype of ALL helps the oncologist guide the recommended treatments. Some are known to respond to chemotherapy and radiation therapy (both to be discussed in more detail in a later chapter) in different ways, so therapies are tailored more to the individual subtype of leukemia. T-cell ALL as a group is historically somewhat harder to treat than the other forms.

When children are diagnosed with leukemia, they have other special studies performed on the abnormal blast cells. Specifically, genetic testing is performed. It is important to know that this genetic testing is not representative of the *child's* true genetic makeup; it is reflective of the genetics inside the *leukemia* cells only. Physicians and researchers have learned over the years by testing the genes in the leukemia cells for thousands of children with ALL that certain groups of children have a better or worse long-term survival based on the leukemia cells' genetics. The reason for this is not always clear. It may have to do with an effect on proto-oncogenes and tumor suppressor genes (discussed in Chapter 1) that get altered within the leukemia cells themselves. Certain genetic markers, such as trisomy (triple copies) of genes 4, 10, and/or 17, and translocations (switching) of some genes such as TEL/AML mean a better prognosis for the child. Other genetic changes, such as the Philadelphia chromosome, which is another translocation or switching between genes 9 and 22, mean a worse prognosis for the child.

There are some genetic changes within specific children that make them more susceptible to having leukemia. The most well-known of these is Down syndrome, otherwise known as Trisomy 21 (the child has three copies instead of the usual two of the 21st chromosome). Children with Down syndrome are much more likely to get ALL than other children, and they are often on monitoring programs through their primary physicians to pick up leukemia cells before the signs and symptoms have time to take hold.

ALL in general has long-term survival rates of about 80 percent. This includes people in all subtypes and all risk groups. The survival rates are higher for some subgroups, and lower for others.

Treatment for ALL mainly involves chemotherapy. Chemotherapy is given in many different forms: intravenous (IV) therapies, muscle injections, oral medications, and intrathecal treatments (given directly into the spinal fluid). This treatment course consists of many phases, and extends to between two and three years of therapy for most children. The most intense treatment is typically given in the first few months. During this time, patients are more likely to have to stay as an inpatient in the hospital to receive their chemotherapy and other medicines. Most of the time, leukemia cells become virtually undetectable after the first few weeks of therapy. However, experience has shown that if treatments are stopped too early, leukemia cells will return and are often harder to fight the second time around. As the treatment continues over time, the intensity of the treatment goes down, and the children receive most of their treatments as outpatients in the clinic or at home. They are still seen in the clinic quite frequently, usually every two to four weeks.

Children who have leukemia cells in the spinal fluid or testicles will usually undergo radiation therapy to these localized areas. Other children who are thought to be "high-risk" for certain reasons may also require radiation therapy. (Radiation therapy is discussed in more detail in another chapter, but essentially involves beams of radiation similar to those in regular X-ray studies, only much more intense, entering the body through the skin and targeting specific areas that need to be treated.) Occasionally, a child may require a bone marrow transplant, usually in instances where the leukemia is not responding as anticipated to the planned chemotherapy or if the leukemia returns after treatment has completed. The major concept behind bone marrow transplant in leukemia is the idea that you can give more intense chemotherapy and/or radiation treatment that is more likely to kill the leukemia cells, while trading out the abnormal bone marrow in a leukemia patient for a more normal bone marrow from another person. (Bone marrow transplantation will also be discussed in more detail in another chapter.)

## Acute Myelogenous Leukemia

Acute Myelogenous Leukemia (AML) is the other type of acute (sudden onset) leukemia that affects children, and it is the second most common form of leukemia in children. It is responsible for 16 percent of all leukemia in children five years and younger and 36 percent of all leukemia between the ages of 15 to 19 years.[2] It's not that AML becomes all that more common in the teenage years; it's just that leukemia in general happens less frequently in this age group, and a higher percentage of the leukemia cases happen to be AML during this time. Similarly to children with ALL, AML causes children to have symptoms of fever, fatigue, and pain. The lymph nodes, liver, and spleen can also be enlarged from infiltration of leukemia cells, but this is usually less obvious than in ALL. AML is less likely to affect the testicles than ALL. Also unlike ALL, occasionally AML cells deposit in the skin, leading to a rash that is actually from the leukemia itself, known as leukemia cutis. Another feature that is unique to AML is the somewhat rare finding of a chloroma (also known as granulocytic sarcoma), which occurs in close to 10 percent of patients with AML. A chloroma is a solid tumor collection of leukemia cells that is not a lymph node. Chloromas tend to be painless and can occur anywhere under the skin on the body. They are often found on the scalp in infants and young children. If biopsied, they show large clusters of leukemia cells that are the same as the leukemia cells in the rest of the body. Occasionally, chloromas appear before any of the other symptoms occur (less than 1 percent of patients); a child can have a chloroma without having any detectable leukemia in their bloodstream.

AML is actually most likely to occur in children under the age of two years. Its incidence continues to decrease between two and nine years of age, then it slowly starts to increase again throughout childhood, adolescence, and adulthood. The overall incidence of AML in children is similar in males and females. AML is quite a different disease in children than ALL. There are certain things in AML that make physicians think that a child is more or less likely to do well with their treatment, but they differ somewhat from the low and high-risk categories of ALL and will be discussed in more detail below.

In ALL, the cell of focus is the lymphoblast. In AML, the cell of focus varies somewhat, depending on what subtype of AML the patient has. There is an older classification of AML that is still used by some called the

French-American-British classification, or FAB. This system assigns a letter-number code to each subtype of AML, going from M0 to M7 (Table 2.1). The basis of this classification is what normal bone marrow cell best resembles the abnormal AML blast cell. As shown in the table, the blasts can resemble cells such as monocytes (a normal white blood cell important in certain types of infection), erythrocytes (the earlier forms of the normal red blood cells that transport oxygen throughout the body), and megakaryocytes (the earlier forms of platelets, which help our body's clotting and bruising mechansisms). The blasts can also be undifferentiated; this means that they are so immature that they really don't resemble any normal cell in the bone marrow. Undifferentiated cells appear in many different types of childhood cancers and are often very difficult to treat. Knowing the specific subtype of the AML blasts helps oncologists come up with optimal treatment plans for the children. For example, M3 AML is very difficult to manage in the first few days to weeks of treatment because of bleeding problems that can occur. However, once a child gets past this initial part of therapy in M3 AML, the overall treatment plan includes a lot more outpatient therapy than other subtypes of AML, and fewer patients require intense treatments such as bone marrow transplants because the overall prognosis is extremely good.

As in ALL, AML patients must also have other special tests performed on the blast cells. Flow cytometry is again used to give the "fingerprint" of the leukemia cell. This information adds to the FAB classification, and in some instances is used instead of the FAB classification to help doctors

**Table 2.1  FAB Classification of AML Cells**

| | Cell Type | Other Features |
|---|---|---|
| M0 | Undifferentiated myeloid cells | Rare form, worse outcome |
| M1 | Minimally differentiated myeloid cells | Common form, average prognosis |
| M2 | Myeloid cells with maturation | Most common type, better outcome |
| M3 | Promyelocytic leukemia | Best outcome, problems with bleeding or blood clots |
| M4 | Myelomonocytic leukemia | Second most common type, average prognosis |
| M4Eo | Myelomonocytic leukemia with eosinophilia | Rare form, better outcome |
| M5a | Monoblastic leukemia | Rare form, average prognosis |
| M5b | Monocytic leukemia with differentiation | Rare form, average prognosis |
| M6 | Erythroblastic leukemia | Rare form, worse outcome |
| M7 | Megakaryoblastic leukemia | Rare form, worse outcome |

determine what types of blasts are present. Genetic testing is also performed on the leukemia cells to give the physicians other information about the best way to treat the leukemia. One specific abnormal genetic finding in AML is something called Monosomy 7. This means that the leukemia cells have only one copy of the seventh chromosome, and unfortunately, this is a predictor of a poor response to usual therapies. Children that have Monosomy 7-related AML are more likely to require a bone marrow transplant for the best chance of cure from the disease.

Certain people are known to be more likely to develop AML than others. These include people with Down syndrome (mentioned above, under ALL). People who have the diagnosis of Myelodysplastic Syndrome (MDS) are also more likely to develop AML. MDS is thought of as a "pre-leukemia" syndrome, and once someone has the diagnosis of MDS they are frequently monitored for the development of true AML. Other exposures have also been associated with AML. These include exposure to a high dose of radiation, such as from the nuclear bombs in Hiroshima and Nagasaki, and exposure to certain types of chemotherapy agents, such as alkylating agents, epipodophyllotoxins, and anthracyclines, all of which will be discussed in a later section.

The survival rate for AML is in general much worse than for ALL. The overall cure rate averaged for the types of AML is just under 50 percent. Teenagers and young infants tend to have lower survival rates, as do people with certain genetic changes to the leukemia blasts such as Monosomy 7. However, certain other genetic changes can lead to a much better overall outcome. For example, M3 AML, otherwise known as APL, has an overall cure rate of greater than 80 percent. Racial background also seems to influence the survival in this disease; children of African-American descent tend to do worse than children from other racial backgrounds. The reason for this is unclear; perhaps children from certain ethnic backgrounds have different genes that either make them more likely to have cancer cells that are harder to treat or make them more resistant to chemotherapy treatments. More work will continue to be done in this area to aid oncologists in giving each individual child the most appropriate therapy for her leukemia.

The treatment for AML can vary greatly, again depending on the subtype of disease. In general, most of the therapy for AML is given intravenously (through an IV) and is more intense than the treatment for ALL, but it occurs over a shorter total period of time. Children with AML often spend month-long blocks of time in the hospital receiving inpatient IV chemotherapy. A good portion of children with AML will require a bone marrow transplant, which is an even more intense form of therapy discussed in a later section.

Children with AML will also require intrathecal chemotherapy (given directly into the spinal fluid) and oral chemotherapy treatments. A child's early response to chemotherapy means a lot for how well they are expected to do long-term. Children who have no visible leukemia cells early in their treatment course are more likely to do better than children who have obvious leukemia still present after the first few weeks of treatment. Oncologists refer to patients that respond quickly to therapy as "rapid early responders."

Another treatment that may happen right after a child is diagnosed is something called leukopheresis. This is done in children who have very high white blood cell counts. These large, sticky, abnormal leukemia cells can clog up their body's smaller blood vessels. A normal white blood cell (WBC) count is between 5,000/uL and 15,000/uL. Children who need this procedure usually have WBC counts greater than 100,000/uL, and sometimes 200,000/uL or higher. Not every child with an extremely high WBC needs to have this procedure. It involves putting a large IV line into the child and attaching the IV line to a large machine called a pheresis machine. The machine is often supplied by the American Red Cross. The machine acts as a filter for the patient's blood; it removes the larger abnormal leukemia cells and puts the more normal cells back into the patient's bloodstream. The procedure usually takes several hours, but it is relatively painless. The only real discomfort occurs when the IV is being placed, but this is usually done in the Intensive Care Unit with the child sedated and under very close monitoring.

## Chronic Myelogenous Leukemia

Chronic myelogenous leukemia (CML) is quite different from the other leukemias that affect children. This type of blood cancer is much more common in adults, and it accounts for only 2 percent of leukemia cases in children under the age of 15 years. It is slightly more common in adolescents between 15 and 19 years of age, making up 9 percent of the leukemia cases in this age group.[3] This chronic leukemia tends to act more slowly and usually has been present for months before it is diagnosed. Sometimes children are found to have this disease on blood tests that are done for non-illness-related doctors visits. While a patient's white blood cell count is usually very high in this disease, there is typically a mild anemia and a normal to even increased platelet count. Because of these lab findings, patients are less likely to have fevers (because their white blood cells are still somewhat functional in fighting infections). They are usually not as tired due to the less severe anemia, and there is less incidence of bleeding because the platelet count is not significantly low.

In this illness, one of the most common childhood complaints is abdominal pain. This pain usually occurs because of a very enlarged spleen. Parents may actually notice that their child's abdomen is distended because the spleen has grown so large. The spleen is an abdominal organ that functions partly in blood filtration; it traps damaged or abnormal blood cells and also helps to destroy certain types of bacterial infections. When children have CML, they often have a high white blood cell count for a relatively long time, and the spleen starts to trap, or sequester, these white blood cells, causing it to grow. In most healthy people, the doctor should not be able to feel the spleen. It sits within the rib cage on the left side of the body near the back. When it enlarges, it starts to grow down towards the pelvis, deep in the left side of the body. It is not uncommon for a spleen to be several times its normal size at the time of diagnosis for CML.

The treatment of CML depends on what phase of the disease the child is in. There are three major phases of CML: the chronic phase (most common phase at diagnosis, minimal symptoms), the accelerated phase (a transition phase where the blast cells are increasing in number), and the blastic phase, or blast crisis (the most severe phase, where more than 30 percent of the bone marrow is replaced by blast cells). The goal of CML treatment is to prevent the patient from ever getting to the stage of blast crisis. Patients are more likely to have problems responding to treatment if the CML has reached an advanced stage. Unfortunately, someone who presents in the chronic phase will progress into the accelerated phase and then to blast crisis if their disease is not treated.

CML therapy has changed significantly over the past few years. The only known *cure* for this disease is bone marrow transplant (the process of which will be discussed in a later section). If the patient has a "match" for their bone marrow (preferably a close relative), then they will receive a bone marrow transplant from that person before their CML reaches one of the more advanced stages. This used to be the treatment plan for all children and teenagers diagnosed with CML. In older adults, oncologists don't always feel that bone marrow transplant is the best option, because it can be more risky in people who are older and have worse health in general. Also, because it can sometimes take years for CML to transform to a more advanced stage, these extra few years in an older adult might be considered enough time. In young patients, however, a few years just aren't enough, and studies have shown that a transplant done in a timely fashion (within one year of diagnosis) offers the best chance for a cure.

However, in recent years, a new medicine called imatinib has been used in the treatment of most types of CML. This medication is a form of chemotherapy. It is a pill that is taken every day, indefinitely, or for as long as it shows effectiveness against the CML cells. CML has a specific chromosome change that is found in most patients' white blood cells. In this case, two of the chromosomes have swapped pieces with each other, leading to a translocation of chromosomes 9 and 22, annotated by t(9;22). This chromosome, otherwise known as the Philadelphia (Ph+) chromosome, is the target of the imatinib therapy. For many patients, this generally well-tolerated medicine can work against CML for several years, keeping patients from going into the more advanced phases of the disease. Unfortunately, because this medicine is so new, it is not known yet if this medicine could work for 10, 20, 30, or even 50 years in these young patients. If it does, this medicine (or another closely related medicine) could eliminate the need for bone marrow transplant in this group. For those patients who do not get an effect from the imatinib treatment or who have unacceptable side effects, most providers would recommend pursuing transplantation for a cure.

# Chapter 3

# TYPES OF CANCER, PART II—LYMPHOMA

## LYMPHOMA

Lymphoma is another major category of childhood and adolescent cancer. It is the third most common childhood malignancy, and it accounts for about 7 percent of cancers in patients under the age of 20 years.[1] Lymphomas tend to be more common in the second decade of life than the first, so they are more likely to affect teenagers than very young children. There are many different types of lymphoma, but most oncologists will categorize them into Hodgkin's lymphoma and Non-Hodgkin lymphoma (NHL). Both groups are cancers of the lymphatic system, which is a part of the body's immune system and includes the lymph nodes, spleen, tonsils, and adenoids. The lymphatic system is present all throughout the body, so these tumors can be present in any part of the body as well.

There are also some similarities between the different types of lymphoma. Any of these patients are likely to present with some amount of lymphad-enopathy (enlarged lymph nodes). Some areas of lymph nodes are easier to find than others, such as in the underarm area (axillae), neck, or groin. Other areas are more difficult to diagnosis, such as the intestinal lymph nodes and mediastinum (middle area inside the chest). Mediastinal lymph nodes can lead to breathing problems because they can partially obstruct the airways in the lungs. Abdominal lymph nodes can lead to abdominal pain and vomiting from obstruction of the intestines. Other common symptoms in lymphoma include fever, significant weight loss, or drenching night sweats, where the clothes and sheets are soaked with sweat and often need to be changed.

In all types of lymphoma, a sample of the tumor tissue is needed to make a diagnosis. In adult medicine, fine needle aspirations (or FNA's) are often done to get a tissue sample for analysis. In an FNA, a needle is inserted into the lymph node to retrieve a "core" biopsy, similar to taking the core out of an apple, but on a much smaller scale. However, in pediatrics this core sample often leads to a lot of confusion about the diagnosis, and it is not recommended.

Most pediatric oncologists prefer to have patients get lymph node excisions, where the entire lymph node is removed for diagnosis. This is helpful because it gives the pathologist a lot of tissue to work with to help with the definitive diagnosis. The lymph node is processed in a specific manner. Some of the tissue can be sent through special machines that look for specific types of white blood cells, and other parts of the tissue are placed on slides that are analyzed under the microscope. The first look under the microscope helps guide other tests that may need to be performed, such as genetic tests or special stains. These special stains can help lead to a diagnosis.

Once the diagnosis is made, the patient has to have another set of special tests to help determine how far the lymphoma has spread throughout the body. These tests may include radiological examinations such as CT (computed tomography) scans and PET scans, and procedural tests such as bone marrow evaluations and lumbar punctures (all of which are discussed in a separate section).

Tumors are staged according to where the disease is located in the body. In general, the lower the stage, the better the prognosis.

Stage I usually refers to a single group of lymph nodes or a single organ affected by the lymphoma.

Stage II usually refers to two or more groups of lymph nodes or a single organ and one or more groups of lymph nodes, but all on the same side of the diaphragm, which is the breathing muscle that divides the chest from the abdomen.

Stage III usually refers to lymph nodes on both sides of the diaphragm affected by the lymphoma.

Stage IV usually refers to lymphoma that has spread to more than one organ other than the lymph nodes, and is a more widely spread disease.

There are some subtle differences in this staging system. These differences depend on the type of lymphoma and the extent of the disease. The health-care provider will discuss these details with the family when the diagnosis is made. Different stages of disease help the provider decide how aggressive to be with the treatment of the lymphoma.

In general, lymphoma is treated with chemotherapy and/or radiation therapy. The details about the types of medicines required, the use of radiation, and the length of treatment will depend on the subtype of lymphoma and the patient's response to therapy. Occasionally, in a disease that is refractory (doesn't respond to treatment) or relapses (comes back after treatment is complete), bone marrow transplantation may be suggested as a form of more aggressive therapy.

## HODGKIN'S LYMPHOMA

*Jason was 10 years old when we learned he had Hodgkin's. His uncle saw him rubbing his neck, and when we asked Jason about it, he said that there were some lumps there. We took him to the doctor to get the lumps looked at, and the doctor said that it was just lymph nodes and that we shouldn't worry about it. She gave him some antibiotics and told us to come back after the antibiotics were done to see if the lumps were any smaller. They didn't get smaller, so then she wanted to do some blood tests and get an X-ray of his chest. She explained to us that she wanted to make sure that there weren't more lymph nodes in his chest. After the X-ray was done, she sat down with us and told us that Jason had a "mass" in his chest, and that she was worried that he had some type of cancer. We were told to go to the emergency room, and Jason ended up getting admitted to the hospital. While we were in the hospital, we met a surgeon who cut out one of the lymph nodes. The doctors told us that it was Hodgkin's lymphoma, and that Jason would have to start chemo fairly soon. [Excerpt of a conversation with a father of a child with Hodgkin's lymphoma.]*

Hodgkin's lymphoma, or Hodgkin disease, accounts for 5 percent of the childhood cancers in the United States.[2] While it can occur in very young children, it typically happens in adolescents. In younger children, boys are more likely to be diagnosed, while among teenagers, girls are more likely to have the disease. The exact cause of Hodgkin disease is unknown, but some think that infections, genetics, and immune system problems may each have some role in the development of this type of cancer.

The most commonly associated virus is Epstein Barr Virus (EBV), also known as mononucleosis (mono). While this virus does not seem to cause Hodgkin's lymphoma, it is found in the tumor cells of almost one-fourth of patients. People who have close relatives with Hodgkin disease may be somewhat more likely to get the disease themselves, but in general the risk is still extremely low. Those who have weakened immune systems have also been found to have an increased risk of developing Hodgkin's lymphoma, but the reason for this is not known.

When the diagnosis of Hodgkin disease is made, the pathologist who reviews the tumor tissue under the microscope determines what subclass of Hodgkin's lymphoma is present. While the details of the subtypes can be complex, most adolescents are diagnosed with the subtype of nodular sclerosing (terms meant to describe the cells seen by the pathologists) Hodgkin's lymphoma. Younger children may have different subtypes, but in general, the treatment remains the same. The only subtype that may receive a somewhat different type of treatment regimen is nodular lymphocyte-predominant Hodgkin's lymphoma, but again, the physicians will determine what type of Hodgkin disease is present before starting any type of therapy.

As in all types of lymphomas, children with Hodgkin disease may have specific symptoms associated with their disease. Some important symptoms include fevers, drenching night sweats, and weight loss of at least 10 percent of body weight. If any of these three symptoms are present, the stage of the disease gets an extra classification of "B" symptoms, while those who are without these symptoms are classified as "A" stages. A person who has a collection of lymph nodes in one area of the neck and no other sites of disease but also has drenching night sweats would be considered a patient with Stage IB disease. The presence or absence of these "B" symptoms affects the overall treatment course for the patient.

Another classification that is sometimes used in patients with Hodgkin's lymphoma is "bulky" disease. Bulky disease refers to a large local group of lymph nodes, which may be harder to treat. The physician determines whether or not the patient has bulky disease before therapy is started. The presence of bulky disease may require a more aggressive treatment plan.

In general, Hodgkin's lymphoma is one of the most treatable cancers in pediatric patients. Children with lower stages of disease have a long-term survival rate of over 95 percent, while those with higher stages of disease have a long-term survival rate of over 85 percent. Overall, the outcome is so good in this disease that most physicians are looking at ways to cut back on therapies to help prevent patients from having significant long-term side effects from their treatment.

All patients with Hodgkin's lymphoma receive some form of chemotherapy, mostly given in intravenous (IV) forms. Patients with more advanced disease often need radiation therapy as part of their treatment plan as well.

## NON-HODGKIN LYMPHOMA (NHL)

*Isaac had been complaining of stomach pain for a long time—usually he was just constipated or wanted attention. But this time was different. He would cry about the pain and I noticed that his belly was getting so big—he looked like a pregnant pre-schooler! I took him to the emergency room, where they examined him, did some blood work, and did a CT scan of his belly. They told me that there was a big tumor in there and that his blood work was pretty messed up. His electrolytes were really high and he needed to get treated for them right away. They sent us to the intensive care unit, and they gave him a lot of fluids and medicines to help fix his electrolytes. The doctor in the ICU said that they were worried about his heart and his kidneys. Then they took a piece of the tumor and found out that it was Burkitt's lymphoma. Isaac started treatment within a day or two with chemotherapy and steroids. We stayed in the hospital for nearly a month. He had to come back to the hospital for more treatments over the next few months, but nothing was as bad as that first time we were there. [Excerpt from a conversation with parents of a child with Burkitt's lymphoma.]*

There are many different types of NHL, but only a handful are commonly seen in pediatric oncology. The three main categories of NHL in pediatric oncology according to the World Health Organization (WHO) are B-cell NHL (Burkitt and Burkitt-like lymphoma and diffuse large B-cell lymphoma), lymphoblastic lymphoma (precursor T-cell and precursor B-cell lymphoma), and anaplastic large cell lymphoma (T-cell or null-cell lymphomas). Each of these types of NHL has differences in its symptoms, treatment, and outcome.

B-cells and T-cells (lymphocytes) are immune cells present in the lymphatic system that serve different functions in fighting infections in the body. As blood cells undergo changes in the bone marrow, developing into leukemia, these B and T lymphocytes can change within the lymphatic system, causing them to become cancerous and grow in an uncontrolled manner. The origin of the first abnormal cell is what leads to the different types of NHL.

## B-cell NHL/Burkitt lymphoma

B-cell non-Hodgkin lymphomas include Burkitt and Burkitt-like lymphomas and diffuse large B-cell lymphoma. Burkitt and Burkitt-like lymphoma account for almost half of the cases of childhood NHL,[3] and this particular type of tumor is one of the fastest growing and most aggressive tumors in children. There are three major types of Burkitt lymphomas—endemic, sporadic, and immunodeficiency-related.

Endemic Burkitt lymphoma occurs mainly in equatorial Africa, where this is the most common pediatric cancer. Over 95 percent of these cases are related to an Epstein-Barr virus (EBV or mononucleosis) infection. It usually affects the facial bones, specifically the jaw.

Immunodeficiency-related Burkitt lymphoma is often associated with immunodeficient states such as HIV (Human Immunodeficiency Virus) infection. Close to one third of these patients have diseases related to EBV infection as well. The most common sites of the cancer include the lymph nodes and the bone marrow. This type is less common in pediatric patients than in adults.

Sporadic Burkitt lymphoma is the most common type of the disease seen in the United States. It is usually located in the abdomen or the neck, and less than 25 percent of these tumors are related to EBV infections.

Burkitt lymphoma in general grows very rapidly. A significant change in the size of the tumor can be noted in day-to-day examinations if not treated. Due to its rapid growth, it is extremely sensitive to treatments that target rapidly growing cells, such as certain chemotherapeutic agents and steroids. Patients that are diagnosed with a large Burkitt lymphoma will often be placed in an intensive care unit setting so they can be watched and treated for a disorder called tumor lysis syndrome. This syndrome is related to the rapid destruction of the tumor cells (lysis, or cell death), and this destruction allows these cells to release compounds into the patient's bloodstream that could be harmful if present in high quantities.

Physicians will monitor patients' electrolyte (such as potassium, phosphorous, and calcium) and uric acid levels very closely. To counteract the rapid electrolyte changes and high uric acid levels, the patients will be given a lot of intravenous hydration. They will also be given medicines selected to treat specific electrolyte or uric acid problems. Occasionally, the patients' kidneys will not be able to handle filtering out these substances as quickly as they need to, so a patient will have to undergo hemodialysis (a mechanical procedure where the blood is filtered through a machine and then returned to the body). Hemodialysis is expected to be short-term (a few days) in the majority of cases, just until the levels of the substances released from the tumor cells have stabilized.

Burkitt lymphoma is usually treated with chemotherapy and antibody therapy. Radiation therapy and bone marrow transplantation are reserved for special circumstances. The treatment is aggressive, but only over a few months. The majority of the treatment is delivered in an inpatient setting. Once a patient gets through the initial concerns of tumor lysis syndrome, the overall cure rate in Burkitt lymphoma is approximately 85 percent.

**Lymphoblastic Lymphoma**

Lymphoblastic lymphoma accounts for almost 20 percent of childhood and adolescent NHL.[4] These lymphomas can be from either a precursor

T-cell parent cell or a precursor B-cell parent cell. Each of these cells has a different function in the immune system, and each type of lymphoma tends to have a different type of presentation. Almost 75 percent of lymphoblastic lymphoma patients have the T-cell form of the disease, which often manifests itself as a mediastinal (chest) mass with accompanying disease in the bone marrow. If there are enough of the abnormal T lymphocytes present in the bone marrow (replacing more than 25 percent of the cells in the marrow), then patients may be given the diagnosis of T-cell ALL, as discussed in the section on acute lymphoblastic leukemia.

Precursor B-cell lymphomas tend to affect the bones or skin, with little effect on the bone marrow. They are related to the precursor B-cell leukemia found in the most common form of ALL, but in a localized form of the disease.

Lymphoblastic lymphoma is typically treated in a similar manner to ALL, with a longer two to three year treatment plan, consisting of IV, oral, intramuscular (muscle shots), and intrathecal (spinal fluid) chemotherapy. As in ALL, the most aggressive therapies tend to be given in the first few months of the treatment plan, with less intense therapy planned for the last several months. When treated with a prolonged course like this, long-term survival for localized disease (stage I or stage II) approaches 90 percent. Patients with more advanced stages of the disease may require some form of radiation therapy, and the overall survival tends to be somewhat lower.

### Anaplastic Large Cell Lymphoma

Anaplastic large cell lymphoma, or ALCL, makes up about 10% of childhood and adolescent NHL.[5] This particular lymphoma can present in many different ways, ranging from skin-only disease, to any lymph node group, to the intestines, and even to the muscle. This form of cancer may progress more slowly, making it somewhat harder to diagnose.

The current treatment of ALCL consists of chemotherapy, given intravenously (IV), orally, and intrathecally (directly into the spinal fluid). The length of therapy is typically from one to two years, and the intensity remains similar throughout the course of treatment. Most are treated with "pulse" regimens, where they are given several different chemotherapy agents at once, given a couple of weeks to recover, and then treated with the same chemotherapy agents again at regular time intervals. Radiation is not a common component of therapy in ALCL. The long-term survival for higher-stage ALCL is somewhere between 60 and 75 percent.

## Chapter 4

# TYPES OF CANCER, PART III—BRAIN TUMORS, NEUROBLASTOMA, AND KIDNEY TUMORS

## BRAIN TUMORS/CENTRAL NERVOUS SYSTEM TUMORS

*When Tashawn was 5, he started complaining of a headache. He would come over to me at times during the day asking for medicine to help his head. For about a week, he would wake up in the morning, and then he would throw up. There wasn't much food in his stomach, and no one else in the family was sick, so I started to get worried. On the day I took him to the emergency room, he was having a hard time walking—he kept falling down and losing his balance.*

*Once the doctors saw him in the emergency room, they found out that he wasn't seeing things very well. He couldn't tell how many fingers they were holding up for him to see. They also said that his eyes looked like they had "pressure" inside of them. They got a CT scan of his head, and they said that it looked like Tashawn had a brain tumor, but they weren't sure, so they'd have to do an MRI test. After the MRI test they sat down with me and told me my baby had a brain tumor and that he would have to have brain surgery.*

*There wasn't a good pediatric neurosurgeon at that hospital, so they sent us by helicopter to another place across town. Once we got there, they put Tashawn in the ICU and told us that he needed to have surgery done as soon as possible because the tumor was causing pressure in his brain. They took him to surgery for several hours. When he came out of surgery, he had all these tubes in him. One was breathing for him, another was giving him fluids, and another was coming out of his head.*

*For the next few weeks he had a hard time walking or talking. It was really hard seeing him like that. They started giving him chemotherapy and then he got radiation therapy. He has been through so much—I just wanted him to have a normal life and be able to play again like he used to. [Excerpt from a conversation with a mother of a child with medulloblastoma.]*

Central nervous system (CNS) tumors are tumors that are present anywhere within the body's central nervous system. The CNS consists of not only the brain, but the spinal cord as well. As a group, CNS tumors are the most common solid tumors in children, and they make up almost 20 percent of all tumors in pediatric oncology.[1] For many parents, this is one of the scariest cancers to be faced with because it is easier for them to picture how changes within the brain could significantly change their child.

CNS tumors are a group of many different types of tumors. They are categorized by the type of tumor cell that is causing the abnormal growth and by the location of the tumor itself. Many people are reassured when they hear the term "benign" in association with a tumor, because they think that benign tumors are not likely to cause significant problems or death. However, any sort of tumor (benign or malignant) within the brain or spinal cord can cause significant changes to the health of the individual, whether it is treated or not. Unlike other cancers in pediatric patients, CNS tumors are very unlikely to spread to other parts of the body such as the liver, bones, or lungs. They are, however, more likely to come back in the same place or another place within the brain or spinal cord.

In adults, CNS tumors are usually tumors that started in another part of the body and then spread to the brain. Examples of these include breast cancer and lung cancer. In pediatrics, CNS tumors are much more likely to be primary tumors of the brain or spinal cord that did not spread from some other site. They are tumors that started from abnormal cells within the neurological system.

The symptoms that occur in patients with CNS tumors vary depending on the tumor location, the age of the patient, and the rate of change that happens within the tumor. Most people think of headaches as being most commonly associated with brain tumors. However, almost all children and teenagers will have a headache at some point in their lives, and naturally, not all of them are associated with brain tumors. Atypical headaches, such as those that are present upon waking in the morning, those that are associated with vomiting, or those that are frequent, recurrent, or progressively worsening, should be taken more seriously.

Other symptoms that may be associated with a CNS tumor include sudden changes in balance, vision, or speech, unexplained weakness in parts of the body, seizures, or significant back or neck pain. Infants may show a bulging fontanelle (soft spot on the top of their head), tilting of their head to one side, or irritability. Teenagers may present with a significant change in their school performance, changes in their growth and pubertal development, or changes in their eating or drinking habits. Of course, a lot of teenagers go through similar changes just because they are teenagers, so it can be difficult at times to tell the difference between normal adolescent behavior and a true medical problem.

One of the most important keys in the evaluation of someone with a suspected tumor in the brain or spinal cord is a thorough medical exam, focusing particularly on neurological problems. The physician will examine the patient's strength, sensation, reflexes, visual movements, balance, gait (how they walk), and their overall appearance before deciding which other studies should be done. The most common radiology studies to look for a brain tumor are CT (computed tomography) scans and MRI (magnetic resonance imaging) scans. CT scans are quick studies that are relatively easy to obtain. However, they are not good at showing specific details, and they may even miss a tumor altogether. An MRI scan is harder to schedule, and the test itself can be quite long. However, when done in the proper manner, they can be used to diagnose almost any type of brain or spinal cord tumor.

When the tumor is found, the next step is to find out what type of tumor it is. Often the doctor will have a good idea of the type of tumor just from the patient's symptoms, the location of the tumor on the MRI, and the particular characteristics of the tumor on the pictures. The best way to make the diagnosis, though, is by getting a piece of the tumor for analysis. A neurosurgeon, who specializes in surgery of the brain and spinal cord, will be consulted to perform surgery. The goal is to remove as much of the tumor as possible without damaging any of the normal brain next to the tumor. Sometimes the location of the tumor is very easy to get to, and a complete resection of the tumor may be possible. Other times, the tumor may be located in an area that will cause significant problems for the patient if the tumor is biopsied, and surgery may not be recommended.

Other tests will likely be done during the evaluation of a CNS tumor. These may include a lumbar puncture or spinal tap (done to look for cancerous cells in the spinal fluid), vision examinations, hearing examinations, neuropsychological testing (similar to IQ testing), and blood tests. The blood tests may be done to check hormone levels, look for specific proteins or markers that may go along with certain types of brain tumors, and check the function of specific organs in the body such as the kidneys.

If a pathologist is able to come up with an accurate histologic (cell-based) diagnosis of the tumor, then the physicians will meet and decide on the best treatment options for the patient. Depending on the type of CNS tumor, this may consist of any combination of more surgery, chemotherapy, or radiation therapy. Some patients require no further treatment and are just monitored closely with scans and physical examinations.

If a histologic diagnosis is not possible because the tumor cannot be biopsied, the physicians will decide on treatment options based on the results of the MRI pictures and the patient's symptoms. Again, treatment may consist of any combination of chemotherapy, radiation therapy, or close monitoring.

There are many different types of CNS tumors, and there are variations within each major category that make classification of these tumors very difficult. Some of the more common types of tumors and broad categories of tumors will be discussed.

### Medulloblastomas

Medulloblastomas make up about 20 percent of pediatric brain tumors.[2] They most commonly occur in the cerebellum or posterior fossa, which is the region of the brain in the back of the head, just above the neck. When a patient has a tumor in the cerebellum, some of the most common symptoms are nausea and vomiting, changes in the vision, and difficulties with balance. Patients are described as "ataxic," meaning that when they walk they almost look drunk.

When evaluating a patient for a medulloblastoma, the physician will check the brain and the spinal cord for other sites of disease. Medulloblastoma can sometimes lead to "drop metastases," where the tumor has spread by "dropping down" into the spinal cord region. Doctors will also check the patient's spinal fluid for signs of disease. Sometimes, they will also look at the patient's bone marrow or bones for other signs of metastatic disease.

Medulloblastomas are treated with surgery, radiation therapy, and often chemotherapy. Chemotherapy tends to be given in an IV format. Patients that have the tumor completely removed by surgery have the best prognosis, and they tend to have a good long-term survival rate in the range of 80 percent. For patients that have metastatic disease at diagnosis, the survival rate drops significantly, and more aggressive treatment options may be sought. Physicians are looking to decrease the total doses of radiation given to children who have good surgical resections and good response to treatment.

## Low Grade Gliomas

Gliomas are tumors that come from a specific cell in the neurologic system, the glial cell. The term "low grade" means that the tumor cells do not appear very aggressive when examined by the pathologist. The most common types of low grade gliomas are juvenile pilocytic astrocytomas (JPA), gangliogliomas, oligodendrogliomas, and some fibrillary astrocytomas. JPAs make up almost 25 percent of pediatric brain tumors.[3]

When a low grade glioma can be completely removed by the neurosurgeons, many physicians will not recommend any further therapy. Close monitoring of the site of the tumor with MRI scans will likely be done, and unless the tumor comes back, no further therapy is needed. If the tumor is completely removed, the long-term survival is greater than 90 percent.

If a low grade glioma is deemed "unresectable" (unable to be removed surgically, for instance a tumor deep in the brain), then chemotherapy is usually given through intravenous and/or oral forms for around 18 months total time. Radiation therapy may also be recommended in these patients, but it is not always used.

## High Grade Gliomas

High grade gliomas also come from the glial cell in the brain. In contrast to the low grade tumors, these tumors are quite aggressive looking when the pathologist examines them under the microscope. The most common types of high grade gliomas include anaplastic astrocytoma and glioblastoma multiforme (GBM). High grade gliomas account for almost 20 percent of pediatric brain tumors.[4]

Patients are evaluated for disease by an MRI of the brain, and sometimes the spine. For anaplastic astrocytomas, an excellent surgical resection can lead to a cure in about one-third of the cases. In GBMs, even with good surgical resection, long-term survival is very poor. There are no good treatments available at this time for GBM tumors with the exception of radiation therapy, but the amount of radiation needed to kill the tumor can sometimes be too harmful for the patient.

## Brain Stem Gliomas

Brain stem gliomas are a special subgroup of glioma brain tumors because of their location. The brain stem is the part of the brain that controls the automatic functions of daily living, such as breathing, blood pressure, and heart beat. When a tumor occurs in this location, no surgical resection is possible.

If a surgeon cut out a tumor in this region, the patient would die from direct damage to the brain stem. In most cases, these tumors are never biopsied, and they are diagnosed simply by their location.

Some physicians have treated patients with brain stem gliomas (otherwise known as diffuse intrinsic pontine gliomas) with focal radiation given directly to the site of the tumor. Others have tried various chemotherapy combinations and medications to stop blood growth within the tumor. There is no known cure for this disease, and typically all children who develop a brain stem glioma will die within a couple of years of their diagnosis. There are very rare exceptions to this rule.

## NEUROBLASTOMA

Neuroblastoma is the most common type of solid tumor (after brain tumors as a group) in pediatric patients. It accounts for 8 percent of pediatric cancers in the United States, and it occurs in the same frequency in boys and girls. Neuroblastoma tends to occur in younger children, usually under the age of five years, and it is rarely discovered in older children or adults.[5] It arises from immature cells in the sympathetic nervous system, which is primarily located in chains along both sides of the spinal cord. The sympathetic nervous system is part of the autonomic nervous system, which controls involuntary (or automatic) actions in the body. It is specifically responsible for signals that people receive during a "fight or flight" response, where they must deal with stressful situations by either fighting or fleeing the offending stimulus.

Primary neuroblastoma tumors can appear anywhere in the body, but most of the tumors appear in the abdomen, usually in the adrenal or suprarenal gland, which is a small gland that sits atop the kidneys. It can also occur as a primary tumor in the chest or neck and can present with metastatic disease in many different places in the body, including the bones, bone marrow, or liver.

*Three months before Sheila was born, we had an ultrasound to look at her growth. The OB doctor told us that there was some kind of mass in her abdomen, close to her kidney, and they thought that it was a neuroblastoma. They didn't tell us much else at that time, just that they would keep doing ultrasounds before and after she was born to see if the mass changed at all. When we went home, we started reading about neuroblastoma on the Internet and we were really shocked to find out that it was a type of cancer. She wasn't even born yet, and she already had cancer? The next few months were scary. Each ultrasound brought new fears and concerns. Thankfully, about three months after she was born, the tumor was gone. I couldn't imagine giving a new baby chemotherapy or some other type of treatment. [Excerpt from a conversation with a mother of a child with neuroblastoma.]*

*Amelia had been complaining that her legs were hurting for about a month. She just seemed more tired than usual. Her Kindergarten teacher said that she didn't play much at recess anymore and complained of the leg pain at school as well. I took her to see the doctor thinking that she probably just had growing pains. He did some X-rays of her legs and drew some blood. Then he said that he wanted to do some special tests on her, where she would have to get an IV and lay still for a couple of hours. He told us that he was worried that she had neuroblastoma, and that it may have spread throughout her whole body.*

*The next few days were a blur. Tests, visits with many different types of doctors. The neuroblastoma was Stage IV. It started in her abdomen and spread to her bones, her liver, and her bone marrow. They told us that she would need to have chemotherapy, surgery, and maybe even radiation treatments or a bone marrow transplant. Her treatments lasted for several months before they said that her disease was in remission. [Excerpt of a conversation with a mother of a child with neuroblastoma.]*

Some believe that neuroblastoma actually comes in two forms: one form that affects children less than 18 months of age and one form that affects older children. When a younger patient presents with a tumor, it is often treated less aggressively and has a better long-term outcome. Most of the patients in the younger group fit into the low-risk or intermediate-risk groups in terms of their therapy, which may consist of just watching the tumor (in the hope that it will self-resolve), surgically removing the tumor, and/or treating the tumor with chemotherapy. Younger infants are sometimes diagnosed with the tumor by prenatal ultrasounds, so the diagnosis is known before they are even born.

Older children tend to present with high-risk disease, often with significant spreading of the tumor to other areas in the body. These children may present with bone pain, fatigue, abdominal distention, and even darkening or swelling of the eyes, depending on the location of the tumor at the time of diagnosis. Some more uncommon presentations are related to hormones that may be produced by the neuroblastoma and include persistent diarrhea, fast heart rate, and fevers.

One specific set of symptoms that is unique to neuroblastoma is the syndrome of opsoclonus/myoclonus, otherwise known as "dancing eyes/dancing feet." These children present with neurologic symptoms related to their body's immune response to the tumor. They may have ataxia (problems with their balance), which may be related to the uncoordinated eye and muscle movements. Children with opsoclonus/myoclonus tend to have high rates of survival with their neuroblastoma, but they may have persistent neurologic dysfunction even after the tumor has disappeared.

The diagnosis of neuroblastoma can be made in several different ways, depending on the presenting symptoms of the patient. One of the simpler ways to test for this disease is through urine studies (ideally done on urine collected for a 24-hour stretch of time). The urine is tested for specific tumor markers called catecholamine metabolites. Specifically, the physicians will test for homovanillic acid (HVA) and vanillylmandelic acid (VMA). Elevated levels of these markers give treating providers an idea that neuroblastoma is present, and it pushes them to search for any signs of tumor.

Another test that is fairly specific for neuroblastoma is a test called an MIBG (metaiodobenzylguanidine) scan, which is discussed in a separate section. This is a nuclear medicine scan that is fairly specific for picking up neuroendocrine tumors, such as neuroblastoma. Other imaging tests that may be done include CT scans, ultrasounds, bone scans, and MRI studies, depending on the location of the tumor. Patients are also evaluated by bone marrow aspirates and biopsies to see if neuroblastoma cells have metastasized to the bone marrow.

Once the tumor has been identified, a biopsy of the tumor will be obtained to confirm under the microscope that it is indeed neuroblastoma. Some other studies will be run on the tissue sample. These studies have significance for the providers as to the treatment of the tumor. These include looking for amplification of a specific gene, called *MYCN*, which is an oncogene that is heavily expressed in most patients with high-risk neuroblastoma.

Other genetic features will be analyzed as well, giving the oncologists more information about how aggressively the tumor needs to be treated. These include changes or mutations in the chromosomes themselves and the DNA index (or ploidy). Normal cells have a DNA index of 1, meaning that they have the normal number of chromosomes present. More aggressive tumor cells have been associated with a DNA index of less than or equal to 1. Other factors that play into how neuroblastoma should be classified relate to histology findings that go along with more aggressive or less aggressive tumors. The histology seen under the microscope is classified as "favorable" or "unfavorable" based on the reading by the pathologist.

All of the factors, including the patient's age at diagnosis, stage of the disease, *MYCN* status, genetic features, and tumor histopathology, play a role in determining whether the patient's tumor is low-risk, intermediate-risk, or high-risk.

Low-risk neuroblastoma patients tend to be younger in age, and they typically have disease that is localized to one area. Biopsy examinations also show good features under the microscope and through genetic testing. These patients are treated with surgery and/or close observation and typically do not need any sort of chemotherapy or radiation therapy. Their long-term prognosis is extremely good.

Intermediate-risk neuroblastoma patients vary in age and they usually have disease that cannot be easily removed by surgery. The characteristics of the tumor when evaluated under the microscope are likely not all good or all bad. Most of these patients will be treated with chemotherapy, often with hopes of shrinking the tumor enough to allow for complete surgical resection. The amount of chemotherapy is often determined by how quickly the tumor responds to the treatment based on lab tests and imaging studies.

High-risk neuroblastoma patients are usually in the older age group and have aggressive features to the tumor cells and spread of the disease to multiple places in the body. These patients require the most aggressive forms of therapy, which include surgery, chemotherapy, and/or radiation or stem cell transplantation. In general, patients with high-risk neuroblastoma have a much worse long-term outlook than those with low-risk or intermediate-risk disease, and most physicians will be very aggressive in their treatment in hopes of the best long-term survival. Unfortunately, these aggressive measures often mean that these children are at risk for significant long-term effects of the same therapy that is used to save their lives from the cancer. Many of these patients may receive treatments that are only available through clinical trials, depending on the severity of the disease and the response to initial treatments.

## WILMS' TUMOR/KIDNEY TUMORS

*When Willie was one and a half years old, we started to notice that his diapers were pink on the inside. We took him to the doctor, and they told us that he had blood in his urine. The doctor also thought that his belly was really full looking, and he thought that he felt something on the left side that shouldn't be there. He sent us to get an ultrasound, and then we found out that Willie had a tumor in his kidney. The tumor was causing the blood in his urine. He had a surgery done to remove the tumor and his kidney. The scar was pretty big, but it healed up very well. The oncologist told us that Willie had Wilms' tumor, which is a type of kidney tumor that is common in kids his age. She said that he would need to get chemotherapy for a few months, and that he should do really well and not have any problems with the tumor coming back again. [Excerpt from a conversation with a mother of a child with Wilms' tumor.]*

Kidney, or renal, tumors that occur in children are very different than the types of kidney tumors that are found in adults. In children, the most common type of renal tumor is Wilms' tumor, which is named after a German surgeon, Max Wilms. Wilms' tumor is one of the more common pediatric tumors, making up almost 8 percent of all pediatric cancers, and is typically found in preschool-aged children.[6] This type of tumor is slightly more common in girls than in boys. It is usually present in only one of the kidneys (unilateral), but occasionally can be found in both (bilateral). Another name for Wilms' tumor is nephroblastoma.

Most children with Wilms' tumors present with a large abdominal mass that is noticed by the child's routine caregiver. Often a story is told that the parent is bathing the child and notices a large hard lump in one side of the abdomen. Other presenting features can be persistent blood in the urine (hematuria), abdominal pain, or persistent high blood pressure (hypertension).

If a physician suspects by her physical exam that a child has a Wilms' tumor, the child will be sent for radiology testing. Often, an ultrasound and a CT scan will be done to determine that the tumor is in fact coming from the kidney. A tumor arising from the kidney in an appropriately aged child is going to be a Wilms' tumor in the majority of cases. There are no blood tests that can diagnose a Wilms' tumor, but some patients may be either anemic, with low blood cell counts, or more rarely polycythemic, with high red blood cell counts. This is due to the production of erythropoietin, a hormone that stimulates the production of red blood cells, in the kidney. Some tumors hinder the production of erythropoietin, and others actually increase its production.

The ultrasound is an important test in patients with Wilms' tumor because it gives the clinicians the best look at the blood vessels coming out of the kidney and their relationship to the tumor. Sometimes Wilms' tumors will extend out of the kidney into the blood vessels in the abdomen, and this can make surgical removal of the tumor more difficult. CT scans of the abdomen give the doctors a good idea about the size of the tumor, any blood that has leaked into the tumor, and any signs of metastatic disease related to the tumor (which, if present, typically occurs in the lungs).

In the United States, patients typically go to surgery prior to receiving any other treatment. During surgery, the surgeon expects to remove the entire kidney (nephrectomy) along with the tumor. Amazingly, most people lead normal lives with only one kidney. The remaining kidney may enlarge somewhat as time goes on to help it compensate for the extra work, but children in general have very few problems related to the nephrectomy. The surgeon will examine the tumor closely for any signs of rupture, because if the tumor breaks open at any time, the patient is treated somewhat more aggressively in the long run. The surgeon will also remove lymph nodes from the abdomen so that they can be examined for spread of the Wilms' tumor in other areas of the abdomen.

After the surgery is complete, the tumor will be sent to pathology for further analysis. The weight of the tumor, the invasion of the tumor through the outer shell of the kidney (renal capsule), and potential lymph node involvement all affect the stage and treatment of Wilms' tumor. The pathologist will also examine the tumor under a microscope for favorable or unfavorable histologic features. Some more aggressive tumors may have something called anaplastic features, which may require more intensive therapy. The pathologists will also examine the tumor for any genetic changes that may make them more aggressive than originally expected.

Very small tumors in appropriately aged patients may not receive any sort of treatment outside of surgery. Other low-staged tumors (Stages I and II) will be treated with intravenous chemotherapy for about four months. Higher-staged tumors and tumors with unfavorable histologic features will typically receive chemotherapy for approximately six months and radiation therapy to sites of the body that have tumor. The majority of patients with Wilms' tumor respond nicely to treatment, and in general the long-term cure rate is approximately 90 percent.

There are some other types of kidney tumors that mimic Wilms' tumor in their presentation but act more aggressively and need different therapy. Such tumors are uncommon, and they are often expected to be Wilms' tumors prior to pathologic diagnosis after the patient has surgery. These include clear cell sarcoma of the kidney and rhabdoid tumor of the kidney. Each of these tumors has a different pattern of metastatic disease, and each needs more aggressive therapy than a similarly staged Wilms' tumor. Patients with rhabdoid tumors of the kidney have a much worse long-term prognosis, with long-term survival rates in the 30 to 40 percent range for lower stages of disease and less than 10 percent for those with metastatic disease.

## Chapter 5

# TYPES OF CANCER, PART IV—BONE TUMORS AND MUSCLE TUMORS

## OSTEOSARCOMA

*Zachary loved to play soccer. He had been playing since he was FOUR years old, and now that he was in high school, he was on the varsity soccer team hoping for a shot at professional play. We didn't think much about it when he started complaining about knee pain. He probably just injured his knee in a game, we thought. But the pain persisted, and he was even having a hard time just walking on it. The team trainer looked at his knee and thought that he should see an orthopedics specialist. The orthopedic doctor got an X-ray of his leg, which showed a tumor in the bone just above his knee. Zachary had to get an MRI to see if it gave a clue as to what type of tumor was there. The tumor had invaded to the knee joint. He was then referred to a specialist who deals with bone tumors, and this doctor did a biopsy of the tumor. They told us that Zachary had osteosarcoma and that he would need some really tough treatments to cure the cancer. He might even have to lose his leg. Our son's focus was on soccer—how could he play soccer if his leg was bad? We just wanted him to survive the cancer. We talked with the surgeons extensively over the next few weeks while Zachary was getting chemotherapy. The surgeons said that they would have to take out part of the bone in Zachary's thigh as well as his knee, and that if he wanted to still play sports it might be best for him to have an amputation. We were amazed at the types of prosthetic limbs that were available. It wasn't easy, but he was eventually able to get back into athletics and even play soccer again after his amputation. [Excerpt of a conversation with a mother of a child with osteosarcoma.]*

Osteosarcoma is the most common bone tumor seen in pediatric cancer. It is usually found in adolescent-aged patients or young adults, but it can also be seen in younger children. The tumor's preference for adolescents seems to go along with the age of growth spurts; those who are undergoing their pubertal growth spurt seem to be more likely to get this tumor than young children or older adolescents. Osteosarcoma tumors are most commonly located around the knee. They will often be located in the tibia (shin bone) just below the knee joint or the femur (thigh bone) just above the knee joint. Other common locations include the upper femur (thigh area), or the humerus bone, which is the arm bone coming out of the shoulder joint. However, this tumor can be found in any bone in the body, including the pelvis, ribs, and skull.

Osteosarcoma is one tumor that seems to have a more definitive genetic association. Genetic changes occur that cause immature, or younger, bone cells to transform into cancer cells instead of normal bone. Patients may have abnormal tumor suppressor genes (discussed in a different section), which make them more likely to develop these types of tumors. There are also some familial cancer syndromes that are associated with young people having an osteosarcoma tumor.

The most common presentation for osteosarcoma is pain in the area of the tumor. Some patients have some minor injury that causes the bone to break at the tumor site, and when the X-rays are done to check out the fracture, the tumor is seen. Patients may also present with a painless mass or swelling in the region.

When a bone tumor is diagnosed, it is usually seen first on plain X-ray studies. There are certain features that the radiologist sees on X-ray that are concerning and make the diagnosis of a malignant bone tumor more likely, but almost all radiologists will recommend a better imaging study to help make the official diagnosis. Often, patients will be referred to have either a CT scan or an MRI done to get a better image of the tumor.

After the tumor has been noted on all the appropriate imaging studies, a biopsy must be performed to confirm what type of tumor is present. For this type of procedure, though, it is critical to have a surgeon skilled in orthopedics, and particularly bone tumors, perform the biopsy. If the biopsy is done in the wrong way, it can contaminate normal tissue and cause the tumor to spread, making treatment more difficult. Following the biopsy, the tumor is analyzed closely under the microscope, looking for certain histologic features that can help with the long-term outlook for the patient.

The different subtypes of osteosarcomas, based on microscopic examination, include osteoblastic (arising from the bone), chondroblastic (arising from the cartilage), fibroblastic (arising from the fibrous tissue), and telangiectatic (arising from certain blood vessels). The telangiectatic forms are much more uncommon, accounting for around 4 percent of all osteosarcomas in these patients. Other determinations about the tumor are based more on the radiologic findings, such as whether or not the tumor is a central tumor (coming from inside the bone) or a surface tumor (coming from the outer surface of the bone). Surface tumors are much more unlikely in children or adolescents, and they are further subdivided into parosteal tumors (low-grade), periosteal tumors (intermediate-grade), and high-grade surface tumors.

Once the diagnosis has been made, the patient will have to have other tests looking for other sites of tumor. One of the more common sites of metastatic disease is the lung, so patients will have a CT scan of the chest. They will also likely have a bone scan and/or PET scan looking for more distant sites of disease.

Patients that have localized disease (no spreading to any other parts of the body) have a much better prognosis than those with metastatic disease. One of the main goals of therapy is to treat the current tumor without allowing it to spread to other locations. The main components of treatment are chemotherapy and surgery.

Chemotherapy for osteosarcoma is almost exclusively intravenous therapy. Patients require several-day stays in the hospital to get their chemotherapy treatments. Common chemotherapy regimens include medicines like methotrexate, cisplatin, and doxorubicin. Patients get chemotherapy for several weeks, hoping to shrink the tumor and kill off most of the cancer cells present before the surgery is done.

The surgical procedure is required to get "local control" of the tumor, meaning that the tumor must be confined and excised from the body to keep it from spreading further. Some patients will require amputations to adequately remove the tumor. Others will have bone grafts put in place of the tumor. The surgeons have to look at the site of the tumor, the size of the tumor, and the expected response to chemotherapy before they make the final decision on which type of surgical removal is required. One of the best prognostic factors for patients with osteosarcoma is the response that the tumor has had to the initial chemotherapy. Patients that have a significant "cell kill," where there is almost no living tumor left, tend to do much better in the long run than patients who have had little response to the chemotherapy.

After the surgery is complete, patients will usually receive more chemo-therapy to prevent further spread of any cells that could possibly remain. Radiation therapy is not typically used in osteosarcoma because it seems to have little effect on the cells, even at very high overall doses. The dose of radiation needed to kill the osteosarcoma is much higher than the normal tissue surrounding the tumor could take.

One special note about osteosarcoma is that it is one of the more common "secondary" tumors found in pediatric cancer patients, meaning that it some-times happens in patients who were treated for some other type of cancer a few years prior. Often, patients will require radiation therapy for their initial cancer treatment, and this radiation puts them at risk for developing these secondary tumors like osteosarcoma. When osteosarcoma occurs as a secondary tumor, it is often harder to treat than if it had been the cancer first diagnosed in the patient. Overall survival rates for patients with osteosarcoma as a primary, or original, tumor are around 75 to 80 percent. Patients with metastatic disease at diagnosis and secondary osteosarcoma in general have worse outcomes.

## EWING'S FAMILY OF TUMORS

*Brittany noticed the lump on her side when she was swimming one afternoon. She asked her sister about it, and her sister brought it to our attention. It wasn't very big, and it didn't seem to bother her, so we didn't think a whole lot about it. A couple of weeks later she mentioned it to us again, and it seemed to have grown. We took her to the pediatrician, and he got an X-ray of her ribs. He told us that there was a bony "lesion" on her ribs and that she should have a CT scan of that area. She got the CT scan of her chest, and it showed a tumor in her rib as well as several tumors in her lungs. The doctors thought that she probably had some-thing called Ewing's sarcoma. She had to go through a lot of chemotherapy treat-ments in the hospital. Her hair fell out, she felt horrible. She also had to have part of her rib taken out and radiation treatments. She's still getting therapy, but she hangs in there. Brittany especially misses getting to spend time with her friends at school, but she is hopeful that she'll be going back to school soon. [Excerpt from a conversation with a father of a child with Ewing's sarcoma.]*

Ewing's family of tumors is a group of cancers that have very similar char-acteristics and are often grouped together under this name. They are made up of Ewing's sarcoma, extra-osseous Ewing's, and primitive neuroectodermal tumors (PNET). These tumors can occur at any age, but they are more com-monly diagnosed in the second decade of life. Most of the tumors occur in the trunk of the body, while one-third of the tumors are found in the long bones of the legs. Ewing's tumors are quite rare in African-Americans, and they are found more commonly in males than in females.

Ewing's sarcoma and PNETs are primary bone tumors, while the extra-osseous Ewing's tumors are soft tissue tumors that can be found anywhere in the body. With any of these tumors, the symptoms are often related to the site of the tumor. In bony tumors, the patient may present with pain at the tumor site. In soft tissue tumors, the patient may present with a tender or non-tender soft tissue swelling. The physician evaluating the lesion will often order radiology studies of the area to get a better sense of what is going on. Basic laboratory studies are not helpful in making the diagnosis of a Ewing's tumor.

Once the mass has been identified through plain X-rays, ultrasounds, CTs, or MRIs, a biopsy must be obtained to get the official tumor diagnosis. As in osteosarcoma, it is better to have a skilled and knowledgeable surgeon performing the procedure to prevent tumor contamination of the surrounding tissues. The pathologist will examine the biopsy specimen and will see certain features that give clues to the diagnosis of a Ewing's family tumor. The cells present are small, round, and blue (some refer to the tumor as one of many types of "small, round, blue cell tumors"). There are also specific genetic changes, or translocations, that go along with the diagnosis of a Ewing's tumor. For instance, the grouping of the Ewing's sarcoma gene, EWS, can usually be found with one of many other genes that are known to be associated with Ewing's tumors. Another clue to the diagnosis of Ewing's is the presence of the CD99 antigen, which is involved in some immune system responses.

After the diagnosis of Ewing's sarcoma or another of the Ewing's family of tumors is made, the patient will have further studies done to assess for any other areas of disease. This will usually include a CT scan of the chest, because one of the more common sites of metastatic disease in Ewing's sarcoma is the lung. Patients will also likely have bone scans, PET scans, and/or MRI studies. Sometimes Ewing's tumors can metastasize to the bone marrow, so patients will have to undergo bone marrow aspirates and biopsies to check for tumor cells.

Certain features of Ewing's tumors have better prognostic features for the patient. These include a location in the extremities, small size of the tumor, age under ten years, female sex, lower levels on some specific blood tests such as lactate dehydrogenase level (LDH) and erythrocyte sedimentation rate (ESR), and localized disease without metastases. With localized disease, survival rate approaches 75 percent; with metastatic disease, the survival rate is much lower, closer to 25 percent.

Treatment of Ewing's tumors involves chemotherapy, with most patients also receiving surgery and/or radiation therapy. As in osteosarcoma, there needs to be good "local control" of the tumor, meaning that the tumor must not be allowed to either spread in the local area or return in the same spot. Physicians will usually give fairly intense intravenous chemotherapy to patients every few weeks for a few months before the local control procedure is attempted. In patients with only one tumor in a site that is easily removed by surgery, they will undergo local control by surgical resection alone. In patients with pelvic tumors or other tumors that are difficult to take out in one block, part of the tumor may be removed surgically with the remaining tumor treated with radiation, or the entire area may be treated with radiation alone. The doses of radiation used for treatment are quite high, and sometimes the normal body structures around the tumor sites will experience problems related to the high amounts of radiation. After the local control therapy is complete, the patient will usually be treated with several more cycles of chemotherapy.

Patients that have metastatic disease need to have aggressive treatment to the metastatic sites as well. Sometimes radiation can be given to these areas, and other times surgical resection can be done. Unfortunately, some patients may be unable to get good local control measures to these lesions, so alternative treatments may be used. In some patients, their physician will recommend an autologous stem cell transplant (discussed in a separate section). In this procedure, the patient is given extremely high doses of chemotherapy and/or radiation to treat the tumor. These doses are higher than the patient's normal bone marrow can stand. The patient's blood counts drop significantly, and they will never recover on their own without intervention. To help treat this problem, the physician gives the patient back some of their own stem cells (which were collected before the treatment) to help the patient's bone marrow recover.

## OTHER MALIGNANT SOFT TISSUE TUMORS

Pediatric and adolescent patients are at risk for developing certain types of soft tissue tumors that can come from one of many different connective tissues of the body, such as muscle, fat, and fibrous tissue. The primary location of the tumor and the primary cell seen by the pathologist when the specimen is examined under the microscope determine the name of the soft tissue sarcoma that is present. These tumors include rhabdomyosarcoma, infantile fibrosarcoma, peripheral nerve sheath tumors, synovial sarcoma, liposarcoma, and alveolar soft part sarcoma. As a group, these tumors make up about 7 percent of all cancers that occur in patients under the age of 20 years.[1]

## Rhabdomyosarcoma

Rhabdomyosarcoma is the most common soft tissue sarcoma, accounting for almost half of all soft tissue sarcomas in pediatric patients. The name means it is a tumor from the skeletal muscle. In can happen in any skeletal muscle in the human body, but the most common sites are parameningeal (close to the base of the skull), orbital (around the eyes), other areas in the head and neck, the extremities, and the genitourinary region (near the bladder, prostate, ovaries, or testes).

The presenting symptoms of rhabdomyosarcoma are related to the location of the tumor. The parameningeal tumors may cause headaches or facial weakness. The orbital tumors may also be related to headaches or eye swelling. Extremity tumors are usually associated with a mass felt within the soft tissues of the arms or legs. Genitourinary tumors may present with a painless mass, unusual bleeding, or difficulty urinating. As in many pediatric cancers, there are no specific blood tests that can help with the diagnosis of rhabdomyosarcoma.

These tumors are usually found by ultrasound, CT scan, or MRI. Once the tumor has been located, a surgeon will either remove the whole tumor or take a biopsy of the lesion. The pathologist will examine the specimen under the microscope, looking for specific histologic patterns that go along with the diagnosis of rhabdomyosarcoma. Two major patterns prevail in this type of cancer: embryonal, which is the most common and has the better prognosis, and alveolar, which is usually associated with higher likelihood of metastatic disease and worse response to treatment. A specific subtype within the embryonal group, found in some vaginal, bladder, or nasal specimens, is botryoid ("grapelike"), which carries a slightly better overall prognosis.

In alveolar specimens, the pathologist will also look for specific genetic changes called translocations, which can occur in the tumor tissue. In these translocations, two separate chromosomes break and reattach to each other. In alveolar rhabdomyosarcoma, the two most common changes are a translocation between chromosomes 2 and 13 (annotated t[2;13], has a worse prognosis) and 1 and 13 (annotated t[1;13], may have a better prognosis). Like Ewing's tumors, rhabdomyosarcoma is another of the "small, round, blue cell tumors" that the pathologist must examine carefully before making a definitive diagnosis.

Once the tumor has been diagnosed, the patient will have radiology studies done to determine the extent of the tumor in their body. Studies for evaluation may include CT scans, MRIs, bone scans, and bone marrow aspirates and biopsies. Once the extent of the tumor has been noted, the physician will work on staging the patient to come up with the most appropriate treatment plan. For rhabdomyosarcoma, this is a complex process, and it takes into account many different features of the disease. The patient is given a "group" number, which is related to the amount of tumor remaining after a surgical resection has been done, ranging from Group I (all known tumor resected, no lymph node involvement) to Group IV (metastatic disease). The patient is then "staged," based on the location of the tumor (some locations are more favorable than others), the size of the tumor, lymph node involvement, and metastatic disease. Stages range from 1 (favorable site without any metastatic or lymph node involvement) to 4 (metastatic disease present).

After the patient has been given a Group and a Stage, he or she is further categorized into a risk classification. Low-risk patients have a good histologic pattern, low stage, and any of the lower group levels. High-risk patients have any histologic pattern and metastatic disease. Intermediate-risk patients are all of those in between. The risk classification is what determines how the patient will be treated. The treatment in general consists of chemotherapy, surgery, and sometimes radiation therapy, with the entire treatment plan lasting a few months to a year, depending on the extent of disease. Chemotherapy is usually intravenous therapy.

Certain factors lead to a better overall outcome in general for patients with rhabdomyosarcoma. These include lower stage or group of disease, more favorable tumor sites (such as the orbit, the head and neck, or the bladder), embryonal histology, age between one and ten years, and no metastatic disease. In the majority of patients, the overall outcome for rhabdomyosarcoma is a 70 percent long-term survival rate.

### Other Soft Tissue Sarcomas

Most other types of pediatric and adolescent soft tissue sarcomas have been grouped into one category: non-rhabdomyosarcoma soft tissue sarcoma (NRSTS). NRSTS make up around 4 percent of all pediatric cancers in the United States as a group, so it has been extremely difficult to come up with more individualized treatment plans based on each specific tumor type.[2] The NRSTS group encompasses many different types of soft tissue sarcomas. They include tumors of fat (liposarcoma), fibrous tissue (myofibroblastic sarcoma, hemangiopericytoma, etc.), smooth muscle (leiomyosarcoma), vascular tissue (angiosarcoma, etc.), cartilage (mesenchymal chondrosarcoma, etc.), and other uncertain sources (alveolar soft part sarcoma, desmoplastic small round cell tumor, etc.). This group also includes malignant peripheral nerve sheath tumors, embryonal sarcoma of the liver, and unclassified soft tissue sarcomas.

The pathologic diagnosis of these tumors can be very difficult to make, and oftentimes the specimens will be sent for second and even third opinions before a diagnosis is given. It is important to have a diagnosis set prior to starting any therapy, because there are times when a slightly different diagnosis can greatly affect treatment. Many different factors will go into the appropriate treatment for the patient: the location of the tumor, any metastatic spread, whether or not the tumor has been completely removed by surgery, the pathology subtype of the tumor, and the anticipated aggressiveness of the tumor.

In general, for lower risk tumors, surgery may be the only treatment required. However, if the tumor has a greater risk for spreading or recurrence, or if the surgeon had to leave some tumor behind, chemotherapy and/or radiation therapy may be recommended. When chemotherapy is used, it tends to be intravenous treatment. Often, the chemotherapy may allow the tumor to shrink enough so that it can be completely removed surgically. Typically, lower risk tumors tend to have a better long-term prognosis than those that are viewed as more aggressive, and metastatic disease also leads to a worse overall outcome for these patients.

# Chapter 6 ❦

# TYPES OF CANCER, PART V—RARE PEDIATRIC CANCER DIAGNOSES
❦

## RETINOBLASTOMA

Retinoblastoma is an eye tumor that occurs in young childhood (infants and children under the age of five years). It is rare and makes up about 3 percent of all pediatric cancers.[1] There are a couple of different forms of the disease, related to the genetics of the patient who develops retinoblastoma. Some patients (40 percent) have something called a "germline" mutation for having retinoblastoma develop. This means that they have a specific change to a chromosome in their body that predisposes them to getting retinoblastoma. This retinoblastoma gene (RB1 gene) is found on the thirteenth chromosome, and it is passed on from parent to child in an autosomal dominant fashion. This means that you need only one abnormal gene to get the disease, and each child of a parent that has this gene has a 50 percent chance of inheriting the RB1 gene as well. Many children found to have the germline mutation were being closely monitored for the development of retinoblastoma because their parent also had the diagnosis as a child.

Other patients have a "sporadic" form of retinoblastoma, which is not related to any specific genetic abnormality. Patients with sporadic disease tend to have unilateral retinoblastoma (only one eye affected), while patients with the germline form may have unilateral or bilateral disease (both eyes affected). All children with bilateral disease are noted to have the germline form of retinoblastoma, and thus are at risk for passing on the disease to their children as well.

The diagnosis of retinoblastoma is often picked up by the pediatrician during a routine "well child" visit. When the pediatrician is shining the light of the ophthalmoscope into the eyes of the infant, he is often looking for the "red reflex" of the eye. This red reflex is actually a red color that is reflected from the back of the eye through the pupil back to the doctor, similar to the "red eye" appearance in some photographs. In retinoblastoma, this red reflex is not present, and the eye actually gives a white look to the back of the eye. This difference can also be seen in certain flash photographs and in the appropriate light setting by parents at home. Other symptoms include abnormal crossing of the eye, poor vision, and an enlarged pupil.

Most children with retinoblastoma have disease that is localized to the eyes. There is, however, a syndrome called "trilateral retinoblastoma" where the patients have disease in one or both eyes and in the brain as well, so most patients with the germline form of the disease will have an MRI or other imaging done of their brain prior to getting therapy. Disease that is localized within the eyes has a very good long-term survival rate of more than 90 percent. Unfortunately, disease that has spread outside the eye has a long-term survival rate of less than 10 percent, so diagnosing the disease as early as possible is key for these patients.

The treatment for retinoblastoma depends on the degree of tumor spread. The goals of treatment are to get rid of the tumor while preserving as much vision as possible, and to also keep patients from having significant long-term effects from their treatment. The classification system used for staging patients with retinoblastoma is evolving, but the stage or group that the patient's tumor falls into determines the therapy that he will receive.

For unilateral tumors that are within the eye, the options for treatment range from enucleation (surgery to remove the eye and the tumor together) to radiation to cryotherapy (freezing of the tissue) to chemotherapy. In unilateral disease, most often the tumor is so large that surgical removal is the only real option. However, in cases where sight may be preserved, clinicians tend to look at the other forms of therapy, such as cryotherapy, radiation therapy, or chemoreduction (done to reduce the size of the tumor, making other treatments more successful). When chemotherapy is used, it is usually given via an intravenous form.

For bilateral tumors, the old treatment was to enucleate, or surgically remove, the eye with the worse disease. However, more recent treatment has been to give radiation and/or chemotherapy and smaller scale surgical treatment to the local tumor in the eyes. Each child has a different amount of tumor when they initially present, and all factors about their sight will be taken into account prior to starting therapy.

One of the most important things for these patients is close follow-up. Patients with sporadic tumors need to have routine follow-up for several years after the diagnosis. Patients with germline tumors also need to have routine follow-up for recurrence of the retinoblastoma, but they also need to be aware that they may be at risk for some other types of cancer later in life. Of patients with germline forms of retinoblastoma, up to 25 percent of non-irradiated patients and 55 percent of radiated patients will have some other form of secondary tumor by 50 years after the diagnosis of retinoblastoma. This risk seems to be related to the RB1 gene that is present in these patients. Also, relatives of patients with germline mutations need to be closely watched for development of retinoblastoma. New siblings of these patients should be screened routinely, and all who are known to have the germline mutation should be screened for retinoblastoma every two months for the first couple of years of life and followed at least yearly thereafter.

## LIVER CANCER IN PEDIATRIC PATIENTS

Hepatoblastoma and hepatocellular carcinoma are the two most commonly encountered liver tumors in pediatric and adolescent patients. Both diseases together account for 1 to 2 percent of all pediatric cancers, and the two diseases are very different from each other. Hepatoblastoma generally occurs in infants or young children under the age of two years, while hepatocellular carcinoma (HCC) tends to occur in younger adolescents.[1] The symptoms of the cancer depend a lot on the age of the patient at the time of diagnosis.

### Hepatoblastoma

Hepatoblastoma seems to form from immature liver cells, and it is usually noted at an early age. The incidence of hepatoblastoma has increased quite a bit over the last 20 or 30 years, and while the cause of this increase is not certain, some think that the increased number of premature infants of very low birth weight are contributing to the increase in hepatoblastoma. There are also some genetic conditions that are associated with a risk of getting hepatoblastoma, which include Beckwith-Wiedemann syndrome and Familial Adenomatous Polyposis.

Patients with hepatoblastoma often present with a significantly enlarged liver. When imaging of the liver is done (ultrasound and/or CT scan), a large liver mass may be noted. Rarely in hepatoblastoma are several liver masses seen. A CT of the lungs is also done because the lungs are the main site of metastasis from hepatoblastoma. Clinicians will obtain blood work for any patient that has suspected hepatoblastoma. There is a "tumor marker" that can be used for hepatoblastoma, meaning that a certain lab value will be elevated when the tumor is first found and when the tumor comes back later. This tumor marker is called alpha-fetoprotein, or AFP. This is a protein that is made by the immature liver cells that cause hepatoblastoma.

In a child of the right age, with elevated levels of AFP, most clinicians are comfortable with the diagnosis. The best treatment for this disease is surgical resection, where the entire tumor is completely removed. Unfortunately, sometimes the tumor is so large that a total resection may put the child at too much risk, so other treatments are initiated. In some cases, chemotherapy (usually intravenous) will be given to help shrink the tumor, making it more easily removed by surgery. In some patients, chemotherapy does not shrink the tumor enough to allow complete resection, so liver transplantation is recommended for a cure.

There are certain features to hepatoblastoma that seem to give a better chance of long-term survival. These include complete tumor removal, the presence of "pure fetal histology" (the cells examined under the microscope resemble those that would be seen in the liver of a fetus), a rapid decrease in the AFP level, and no metastatic disease at diagnosis. In general, the long-term survival rate with hepatoblastoma is around 70 percent.

## Hepatocellular carcinoma

The incidence of HCC has remained stable over the past several decades. There are, however, certain races that seem to be much more susceptible to developing HCC than others. For example, the incidence of HCC is ten times greater in some Asian countries than it is in the United States. This is likely related to hepatitis B infections. In the United States, children are immunized against hepatitis B. In many other countries, the hepatitis B infection is extremely common, and mothers who also have this disease may pass on the illness to their children during childbirth.

Patients that present with HCC tend to be sick; they often have weight loss, vomiting, abdominal pain, and loss of appetite. They may also be jaundiced (yellow tinting to the skin and eyes). Children may present with a slowly enlarging mass in the right upper area of the abdomen. Patients who have been infected with hepatitis B or C (both viral infections) are more at risk for developing this type of cancer. Other risk factors for having HCC include chronic liver disorders such as biliary atresia (poorly formed biliary tract system), chronic cholestasis (poor movement of bile within the biliary tract system), or glycogen storage diseases (problems with metabolism of certain carbohydrate products). People who have these risk factors have usually already been diagnosed with the other illnesses for many years prior to developing HCC.

As in hepatoblastoma, patients often have tumor markers present. In almost half of the patients, AFP levels will be elevated. Another tumor marker that is often found in HCC is beta-human chorionic gonadotropin (B-HCG), which is the hormone elevated in pregnancy. Imaging studies, such as liver ultrasound or CT scan, will show a more invasive tumor than that seen in hepatoblastoma. The cancer is often multi-focal, meaning that there are several spots of tumor that spread throughout the liver.

Once a liver biopsy has been done, the pathologist will confirm the diagnosis through examination of the specimen. One key feature that may be seen under the microscope is a variation in the tissue histology called fibrolamellar carcinoma. There are characteristic appearances to the cells in patients with this variant, and the fibrolamellar subtype tends to have a better long-term survival in general. After the diagnosis has been confirmed, the patient will have imaging studies done to look for other areas of disease. These often include a CT scan of the lungs and a bone scan.

After determining the extent of tumor, complete surgical resection is the best treatment option. However, only about one-third of patients have a tumor that is easily removed, so often physicians will recommend some form of chemotherapy treatment (usually intravenous) to reduce the size of the tumor, making it easier to remove. Another form of treatment in these patients that has limited use is a practice called chemoembolization, where chemotherapy is infused directly into a branch of the hepatic artery (one of the main arteries for the liver), with the aim of killing off the tumor that is present at the end of that blood vessel branch. Another option for therapy is liver transplantation, but this is only useful in patients who do not have disease in other parts of their body.

As with hepatoblastoma, certain features are associated with a better long-term outcome. These include complete surgical resection of the tumor, rapid reduction in the tumor marker levels, fibrolamellar variant to the pathology, and no metastatic disease. In general, the long-term survival rate from HCC is around 25 percent.

## THYROID CARCINOMA

The thyroid gland is a small gland located in the neck, just below the cricoid cartilage, or "adam's apple." This gland has four parts (two on each side) and is shaped like a butterfly. It is responsible for regulating some of the body's metabolism. Specifically, it helps regulate the body's energy level and its response to weather or temperature changes. Many people have heard of someone having hypothyroidism, where the thyroid gland does not function appropriately. These people often have a hard time dealing with cold weather, they tend to be sluggish, and they often gain weight. Hyperthyroidism is the opposite of this—people tend to be more hyperactive with difficulty sleeping; they are hot in inappropriate situations, and they may lose weight. Occasionally, patients with either of these signs (hypothyroidism or hyperthyroidism), may in fact have thyroid cancer. Thyroid cancer is extremely rare in pediatric and adolescent patients, and it accounts for about 1.5 percent of all pediatric cancers.[2]

Thyroid cancer is usually detected in people without any symptoms, though. Patients may present with a lump in their neck that does not cause any change in the way their body functions. If a lump is noted, the physician will usually recommend an ultrasound of the thyroid gland or neck to see where the lump is located. Sometimes, a nuclear medicine study will be ordered to see if the lump, or nodule, has any concerning metabolic activity. Often, a biopsy of the nodule is done to see if it is in fact cancerous. Most thyroid nodules are not cancerous, and they just need to be watched closely by the doctor's exam and sometimes by ultrasound studies.

When thyroid cancer is detected, the pathologist makes a determination on which type of thyroid cancer is present. The major subtypes of thyroid cancer are based on what is seen under the microscope. They are papillary (70 percent), follicular (20 percent), medullary (10 percent), and anaplastic (less than 1 percent). Each term describes a pattern of cells that is seen by the pathologist, and each has some bearing on the expected overall outcome of therapy. Certain subtypes are also associated with certain genetic diseases that make people more likely to get thyroid cancer or some other forms of cancer, such as medullary carcinoma and sometimes follicular carcinoma.

Once the diagnosis is made, the patient will be taken to surgery to have most, if not all, of the thyroid removed. The surgeon will also often take out several lymph nodes in the neck in regions close to the thyroid to look for spread of the cancer. After the surgery, the patient will develop hypothyroidism and the symptoms that go along with it. A few weeks after the surgery has been done, the patient will have another nuclear medicine study, looking for any functioning thyroid tissue in the body. Based on the results of this study, patients will be given a certain amount of radioactive iodine that can help destroy any remaining thyroid tissue in the body. The dose increases for more widespread disease. Iodine is a substance that is needed for the thyroid gland to work in normal people. The thyroid is really the only part in the body that uses iodine to any degree, so when the radioactive iodine is given, it is effective at destroying only thyroid cells, not harming other parts of the body. This treatment is known as radioactive iodine ablation. Once the patient has stabilized from the treatments, synthroid (a thyroid hormone replacement) is started to treat their symptoms of hypothyroidism. This medication dose can be adjusted based on laboratory thyroid levels and patient symptoms.

The surgical removal of the thyroid and one treatment of radioactive iodine ablation usually leads to an effect in almost 70 percent of patients. Some other patients need additional treatment to go into remission. In general, pediatric patients do very well with good long-term survival rate of 95 percent and relatively few side effects.

## MELANOMA

Melanoma is a skin cancer that affects people of all ages. It used to primarily be considered an adult cancer, but lately its incidence has been increasing in younger children and teenagers.[3] Melanomas are tumors that arise from abnormalities in the cells that give pigment (or melanin) to the skin, eyes, and hair. While it is not the most common form of skin cancer in the United States, it is the most deadly form of skin cancer. Pediatric patients in general, tend to do well with treatment, with long-term survival rates in the 90 percent range.

Certain features put people at risk for developing melanoma. In adults, most think of excessive sun exposure in the past that led to significant sunburns. In children and adults, there are other things that are more commonly associated with melanoma. These include the presence of certain congenital diseases, such as giant congenital nevus (giant mole), xeroderma pigmentosum, and Werner's syndrome. Some children are actually born with melanoma as a result of tumor being passed from the mother to the infant through the placenta. Other features that seem to be associated with melanoma include a history of many moles or atypical moles, and medications that suppress the body's natural immune system.

There are certain features of a mole that make it more likely to be an actual cancerous melanoma. Many people have been taught the "ABCDE's" of melanoma. "A" stands for asymmetry, meaning that if you fold the mole in two, the two halves do not match. "B" stands for border—if the borders or edges of the mole are blurry instead of crisp, then there is cause for concern. "C" stands for color, so any colors other than the typical black or brown are concerning. "D" stands for diameter—if the mole is bigger than the eraser end of a pencil, then it is too big. "E" stands for evolving, so significant change or evolution in the mole can be a problem. If a physician evaluates the skin lesion in question and notes that several of these factors are present, she is more likely to request a biopsy of the lesion for further evaluation.

Once the mole has been biopsied, the pathologist will examine the mole for features consistent with melanoma. If melanoma is present, there are certain features that will affect the overall outcome and treatment of the cancer. These include the thickness of skin involved with melanoma, any lymph nodes that are involved, how quickly the cells are dividing and growing, and ulceration of the site of the melanoma. In general, pediatric patients do better than adults with melanoma, and lesions that are found on the arms and legs are usually more easily treated than other areas.

Melanoma can metastasize to other parts of the body, include the lungs and liver, so physicians will recommend imaging studies to determine if the disease has spread at all. Often as part of the staging workup, the patient will have something called a sentinel lymph node biopsy. This is a procedure where the surgeon wants to find out which lymph node is the first lymph node that would typically be affected if the tumor were to spread. The surgeon will inject a type of dye into the tumor region and follow it to the first lymph node. This lymph node will then be removed, along with several others in the same region, to see if it has any signs of melanoma present. Melanoma can spread through the body's lymphatic system or the blood stream.

The priority treatment for melanoma that has not spread anywhere is surgical removal. The surgeon must remove not only all of the tumor, but anywhere from one to three centimeters of skin around the tumor as well, depending on how much skin thickness is affected by the tumor. There are certain types of intravenous therapy that have been given to help treat melanomas that have spread to areas that cannot be surgically removed, and in certain situations they can be effective therapy. These include the medicines interferon, interleukin-2, and certain chemotherapy agents.

## NASOPHARYNGEAL CARCINOMA

Nasopharyngeal carcinoma is a rare pediatric cancer that occurs in the lining of the nasal cavity and throat (pharynx). In the United States, it occurs at the rate of 1 in 100,000 people under the age of 20 years, but it is somewhat more common in other areas of the world, such as Southeast Asia and North Africa.[4] This discrepancy in frequency is likely related to a virus called the Epstein-Barr virus (EBV), which is the virus associated with infectious mononucleosis. This virus seems to have a role in several different types of cancers, and it is usually associated with nasopharyngeal carcinoma as well. EBV is even detected within the biopsy specimens of this cancer, specifically on the surface of the tumor cells.

Patients that present with nasopharyngeal carcinoma often have symptoms related to their face and neck. They may have facial pain, recurrent sinus infections, throat discomfort, or neck swelling. Neck swelling is usually related to the spread of the primary tumor site. Nasopharyngeal carcinoma tends to spread to lymph nodes in the neck. Rarely, it will spread to other parts of the body such as the bones, lungs, or liver.

Diagnosis is usually made from a tissue biopsy obtained from the primary site in the throat or nasal cavity. Usually, patients will have some sort of endoscopy procedure done (where a long thin tube with a camera attached is inserted in the nose or throat) to actively see the area involved. Once the diagnosis has been confirmed by pathologic evaluation of the biopsy specimen, patients will undergo studies to see if and where the tumor has spread. These studies may include CT scans, MRI studies, bone marrow aspirates and biopsies, and nuclear medicine studies such as bone scans or PET scans.

Most patients have an advanced stage of disease at the time they are diagnosed, with spread of the tumor to the neck region. It is rare for patients to have true distant metastatic disease when they are first starting treatment. Long-term survival in nasopharyngeal carcinoma ranges from 80 percent for patients without spread of their disease to 40 percent for patients with more advanced disease, and even lower for those who actually have true metastatic disease at diagnosis.

In general, the tumors in nasopharyngeal carcinoma are very hard to remove surgically, so very few patients have surgery as their form of "local control." Most patients are treated with intravenous chemotherapy and high dose radiation therapy to control and hopefully cure their disease. Unfortunately, the doses of radiation are so high that they tend to have significant side effects for the patients. Often, because the radiation is done in areas that affect eating and drinking, some doctors will recommend the patient have a feeding tube surgically inserted through the skin of the abdomen, directly into the stomach so that they patients can stay well-nourished during their treatment.

## GERM CELL TUMORS

The term "germ cell tumor" refers to one of many potential tumors that come from cells that migrated to the gonads during embryo formation. This migration occurred in the midline of the embryo, so these tumors tend to be present in the middle of the body, such as the inside middle of the chest (mediastinum), middle of the abdomen next to the spine (retroperitoneum), and the middle of the lower back and pelvis region (sacrococcygeal). They also occur in the gonads themselves (testes in the male, ovaries in the female). As a group, germ cell tumors account for almost 4 percent of all pediatric cancers.[5] However, there are many different variations of the germ cell tumor included in this group, and the identification of the subtype of these tumors can be quite complex.

Germ cell tumors can be malignant or benign, depending on the specific subtype of the tumor. The malignant tumors include tumors such as choriocarcinoma, yolk sac tumors, and immature teratomas. Benign germ cell tumors include mature teratomas. The benign or malignant characteristics of the tumor can change the type of treatment given.

When a patient presents with a germ cell tumor, the symptoms are related to the location and size of the tumor. Females with a gonadal germ cell tumor will present with a lower abdominal mass. Males with a gonadal germ cell tumor will present with a testicular mass. Some children present with masses in the lower pelvis or spine, or they may present with respiratory symptoms related to a mass in the chest.

Once the tumor has been located, the physicians will arrange for either a biopsy or complete surgical removal of the tumor. The pathologist will then examine the specimen very carefully for certain cell types under the microscope. There are many different types of cells that can be present in germ cell tumors, and it is very important for the pathologist to look for the most aggressive types of cells that may be present. Unfortunately, germ cell tumors are often quite large when they are removed, which makes analysis of the entire tumor nearly impossible. In most cases, the oncologist will treat the patient based on the worst type of cell present (the cell with the most malignant potential).

The physicians will also order blood tests for the patient to look for "tumor markers," which are elements in the blood that are associated with certain types of tumors. As the levels of the tumor markers fall, the physician can know that the tumor is being treated appropriately. Tumor markers commonly found in germ cell tumors are alpha-fetoprotein (AFP), and beta human chorionic gonadotropin (B-HCG, the pregnancy hormone).

When these tumor markers are present in any amount, the oncologist is more likely to treat the tumor as malignant, no matter what the pathology specimens show, because the tumor markers are associated with only certain types of malignant histologic features.

Certain features about germ cell tumors make them easier to treat. These include locations in places other than the chest, benign mature teratomas, patients younger than 15 years of age, and patients who have no signs of metastatic disease at diagnosis. The physician will take these features into account when recommending specific types of potential treatment for patients with germ cell tumors. If metastatic disease is present, it will often be located in the lungs, liver, or bones. The general outcome for pediatric patients with germ cell tumors is very good, with long-term survival rates above 90 percent.

The major part to the treatment of germ cell tumors, malignant or benign, is surgical removal. In some instances (such as boys with testicular tumors that are completely removed), even if malignant cells are noted by the pathologist, the physicians may recommend surgical removal with only close follow-up examinations. In others, the concern for tumor recurrence is so great that intravenous chemotherapy will be recommended for various lengths of time depending on the subtype, response, and location of the tumor. Sometimes, radiation therapy is recommended as well, but this is less frequent than chemotherapy.

# Chapter 7

# TELLING THE CHILD

How do you tell a child that she has cancer? It's hard enough to tell an adult about this complex and life-threatening illness, much less a child or teenager. Most adults and many adolescents know something about cancer. They know that it is a medical diagnosis, and a lot of times they associate it with death. People who hear the word "cancer" look back on their own experiences—maybe an older family friend or close relative had some form of cancer. Hopefully their past experiences with others who had this disease were fairly positive, but in many cases, especially with older adults, cancer leads to suffering, many medical treatments, and even death.

The adults in charge have to think about the individual child and decide what information they feel is appropriate to share. Most medical professionals in this situation would advocate telling the child (in an age-appropriate manner) as much as possible about his illness and what it will change in his life. It is very difficult to hide things from these young patients. Even toddlers will pick up on stress around them, and each child or adolescent will handle this stress in a different way.

In most instances, physicians provide information directly to the parents, but often the child will be present in the room when this information is given. This can be difficult, especially in the case of elementary school-aged children, because they will hear a lot of unfamiliar words and pick up on verbal or non-verbal cues from their parents that make them realize they are sick. Some children may even assume that they are going to die, particularly if they have heard these same types of words used in the context of older family members who later passed away. Parents and physicians alike need to be sensitive to the patient and make sure that he understands to the best of his ability what is happening to him.

Again, most healthcare professionals would recommend letting the child know about her diagnosis and upcoming treatments from the very beginning. There is a possibility, however, that a parent might give the child misinformation that could affect her trust in others. For example, telling your child that she will be able to get most of her cancer treatment at home or in the clinic, only to find out that she actually has to be in the hospital for months at a time. This will hurt the child's trust in the adults around her and will make future discussions about her treatment and illness very difficult. Open communication among the parents, healthcare workers, and young patients should start even before the diagnosis is made, when the patient starts having tests to determine whether cancer is present.

When communicating a serious medical illness to a child, the parents and providers must take into account the child's age, developmental level, and ability to understand. Naturally, you don't talk to a teenager the same way you would a toddler. It is very important to put the diagnosis of cancer into a context that each patient can understand. Once children understand that they have cancer, caregivers must also understand that each child deals with difficult information in different ways. Some will internalize their feelings, while others may act out in anger towards others. Much like an adult goes through different stages of acceptance, so will a child or an adolescent.

## INFANTS AND TODDLERS

In general, infants and toddlers aren't going to understand anything that you tell them about the diagnosis of cancer. They will, however, pick up on the emotions and the actions of those around them. They depend on structured routines to help them feel safe. While you can't explain to them why they have to be put through all these tests, you can support them by showing them affection and doing everything within your power to stick as close as possible to your usual routine. Of course, this is oftentimes easier said than done in the hospital setting, where it's almost impossible to get a period of uninterrupted sleep, and it seems like every time you turn around someone else is in the room wanting to talk to you or take your child's blood pressure or perform a blood test.

*When Destiny was being treated for rhabdomyosarcoma, she spent a lot of time in the hospital. She had to come to the hospital every few weeks to get chemotherapy. Every time we went home from the hospital, I had to struggle to get her back to her usual routine—she would wake up at all hours of the night, her feeding schedule was off, and she had to be held constantly. I finally learned to work with the hospital nurses to help her stay "on schedule" while she was getting chemotherapy. This meant putting a sign on the door when she was sleeping to minimize disturbances, getting her blood tests sent later in the morning, and cutting back on how often they messed with her in the middle of the night. Most of the hospital staff was really helpful in making this happen. After we were able to work with Destiny's schedule in the hospital, it was much easier dealing with her at home in between chemotherapy treatments. [Excerpt from a conversation with a mother of a child with rhabdomyosarcoma].*

When dealing with these very young patients, parents should discuss the hospital care with the doctors and nurses to help keep their child in some sort of routine. Perhaps the middle of the night vital signs can be skipped under certain circumstances, or maybe the parent could request that the doctors do their rounds a little later in the morning to let their infant maintain a better sleeping pattern.

## PRESCHOOL-AGED CHILDREN

Preschool-aged children usually don't mind going to see the doctor. Some are often excited about the visit to the doctor's office and ask a lot of fun questions about what they'll get to do during their appointment. That enthusiasm and excitement quickly fades, however, when the child is seeing the doctor to undergo an evaluation for cancer. Often, these children have been sick for quite a while and show little reaction during the initial consultations, other than the typical crying with blood draws or other uncomfortable procedures. However, when they start to feel better, they start to ask questions.

Keep in mind that even though these children may have been very sick, they were still able to gather some information from the people around them. They may have seen Mommy and Daddy crying or even arguing about things that have been going on. They may associate certain people with their parents' frustration. Take, for example, the physician who comes to give the parents the latest updates on the child's health. The young child may only know that every time "that person in the white coat" comes to talk to his parents, they cry. That makes the physician the "bad guy" in the eyes of the child.

Explaining the diagnosis of cancer to someone this young is extremely difficult. Some parents will avoid using the word "cancer," but sometimes the child will hear this word from someone else who is helping in his care and become quite confused. Many people will change the terminology with children of this age. They may tell the child that he has some kind of sickness inside them that the doctors and nurses are going to make better; but it's difficult to explain to a child this age that the very things that are supposed to help them will actually make them hurt, throw up, change the way they look, or make them generally feel sick.

Preschoolers need to be told the truth about what's going on and what's happening to them. If something is about to happen that will probably cause the child some pain, parents and providers should not tell them that "this won't hurt." Lying to children to make them cooperate is not helpful.

Preschoolers also need to know that they are not the ones in charge. Once a young child gets diagnosed with cancer, people may start to treat them differently; perhaps they will let them get away with staying up late at night, or maybe they will get to pick out presents every time their parents go to the store. Discipline and order are very important in this age group. These children need to stay on a routine schedule as much as possible, and they need to understand that their parents are still in charge.

> *Caroline was almost two when we found out she had leukemia. She really was a sweet and loving child, but when she was sick she just cried all the time. I was surprised at how she treated the doctors and nurses taking care of her. She didn't get mad at them—she just ignored them! Every time someone else walked into her hospital room, she closed her eyes. She figured out that if she was "sleeping," people usually left her alone. Sometimes she would open her eyes just a bit to make sure that the outsider was gone before she started watching TV or talking to me. [Excerpt from a conversation with a mother of a child with leukemia]*

Many children this age will try to ignore the people who are taking care of them. Some children are much more blatant in their actions toward non-family members. It is not uncommon to have the child disappear under the covers or yell and scream when approached. With time, however, these children will warm up to the healthcare providers and will actually accept the things going on around them as "normal," probably much more so than their adult caregivers ever will.

## ELEMENTARY SCHOOL-AGED CHILDREN

Elementary school-aged children have a better understanding of the more complex medical issues and treatments that are surrounding them, but they tend to worry more about others around them and how their illness will affect the way others treat them. Parents should be up front with these patients about their diagnosis and the upcoming treatments, but they should also realize that for some children you can give too much information.

By this age, many parents are aware of how their child handles stressful situations. You have the child who gets a small scrape or cut and becomes very emotional, and then you have the child who may suffer a broken bone during a sports game and want to go right on playing. Gauging a child's reaction and response to certain circumstances and situations will help in making her feel more comfortable with the tough road ahead. In addition, the parents' attitude about the current situation will greatly influence the child's perspective on how to react.

Friends and classmates start to become an issue for this group. The child will probably worry a lot about what his friends are going to think about him if he loses his hair or has to undergo some major surgery that will change his appearance. Even a child who loved going to school before may attempt to avoid any contact with the school, his classmates, and his friends while he's sick or undergoing any treatments. It is often helpful to contact one or two close friends early on in the diagnosis and treatment process. Speaking with the parents of these children and explaining the current situation may make things easier for a visit with a close friend. If one or two trusted friends accept the changes in the patient and continue to treat him as they always have, then the child may feel more comfortable about seeing more people out in public or in the school setting.

Many children can actively attend school during their cancer therapy. Most parents also arrange for at least a partial homebound schooling process, in case the child doesn't feel well enough to attend school for any significant period of time. Many hospital treatment centers will have school teachers who help teach children who have to remain as an inpatient for any real length of time. Others allow the homebound schooling team to see the children in the hospital to continue their studies.

When a child does return to school, many of the classmates will have a lot of questions and maybe even concerns about the child's illness. Most pediatric oncology centers can send someone to the school to help educate the other children about the patient and about the cancer they have. Children will wonder things like "Can I catch cancer?" and "Did they do something bad to get cancer?" Clearing up these misconceptions from the beginning can be very helpful in ensuring that the patient is able to return to a more normal environment from the beginning.

*We always enjoy visiting the elementary schools of our cancer patients. Sometimes we meet with individual classes, and sometimes we give presentations to the entire school. Most of the time, we give a brief talk about the type of cancer that the student has and ways that the cancer affects the student. If the setting is appropriate, we may show the students a video about what's going on. Then we turn to the children for questions. You never know what the children may ask. We encourage any question, though, because if children think that they're going to be made fun of for a silly question, they'll just sit there and worry. Occasionally, the student likes to show the classmates the central line or how they get shots. Most of the other kids think that this is really cool, and it helps the patient feel extra special. [Excerpt from a conversation with a nursing group from a Pediatric Oncology Center].*

As is the case for younger patients, maintaining a routine for these children is important. Setting age-appropriate guidelines for how they should behave and treat others is also a vital component to their care. Discipline must be maintained, and just because a child has cancer or is sick does not mean that the child has free rein and can do whatever she wants to do. After being diagnosed with cancer, many parents and other family members will start to spoil a child in this age group. While it is nice for the child to know that people are thinking about her and doing things for her, it can be detrimental to her future if she starts to get everything she wants just because she is sick. This is a difficult balance for parents and caregivers, to keep things as normal as possible despite the fact that a life-altering event has just taken place.

## ADOLESCENTS

Teenagers are going to understand the most about what is happening to them, and they will seem to understand more about cancer than their younger counterparts. However, they can have some of the worst problems in coping with the diagnosis of a serious medical illness. Adolescents in general have the goal of being like their peers. Anything that makes them stand out from the crowd can affect their sense of self esteem, and few things make you stand out from the crowd more than having cancer.

Imagine having to deal with all of the normal changes that happen with adolescence—puberty, growth, weight gain, school difficulties, etc.—and add to that a diagnosis of cancer. Hair loss from chemotherapy, body changes and acne from steroids, scars from surgery, and in some patients more severe body changes such as an amputation, can severely affect their peer relationships.

In most situations, adolescents should be treated as adults when it comes to informing them about their illness and treatments. Most oncologists will actually go through the consent process with the adolescent patient, just as they do with their parents. This consenting process in children under 18 years of age is considered obtaining "assent." These older children will do better with their treatment if they understand why they have to have the therapy, how the treatment will be accomplished, and how they have some control over what is happening to them.

However, in some instances, teenagers under the age of 18 will get to a point where they refuse treatment. While it would be ideal to have their approval for the things that are going to happen to them, legally the adult guardian has the last say in how the treatment will be handled. In instances where the patient and the parent disagree about how to proceed, the provider and support staff should attempt to bridge the gap between the disagreeing parties. Often, a psychologist or social worker can help make sure that communication is open and that all involved understand what goes on with the treatment process.

> *David really enjoyed the teen-night meetings at the cancer support house. It was the one place where he could hang out with friends without worrying about being bald or if he needed to take a break and rest. He also enjoyed being able to hear about others' cancer battles—I think it made him feel stronger about his own situation, knowing that he wasn't alone in his fight against leukemia. The other children and teenagers looked up to David and saw him as a source of inspiration because of his attitude about fighting cancer. [Excerpt of a conversation with a father of an adolescent with leukemia].*

Adolescents may benefit the most from age-appropriate support groups. For a teenager, knowing that he is not the only one dealing with such a serious illness can mean so much to his self-esteem and spirit. Usually, the teenager that has a good strong network of friends before the diagnosis will be the one that seems best prepared to handle the physical changes associated with cancer. This doesn't mean that he won't be ashamed or embarrassed about his hair falling out or the skin changes that occur, but it may help him feel less isolated from the "normal" world.

One of the other major problems in teenagers undergoing cancer treatment is compliance. As a parent, you want your child to have some responsibility for her treatment, and an adolescent-aged patient doesn't want to be "babied" by their parents. However, even the most conscientious adolescent has been known to miss medications and even go out of her way to avoid taking things that could be vital to her treatment. Even though an adolescent is smart enough to know better, her developmental stage in life still gives her some sense of invincibility, which can affect the way she thinks about her treatments.

## Chapter 8

# PROCEDURES AT DIAGNOSIS, IN THERAPY, AND AFTER THERAPY

There are many different procedures in which your child may be involved during an evaluation for cancer. These range from simple blood tests to surgical procedures to radiology studies. Having some idea about why and how these tests are performed will allow you to help make your child more comfortable during some scary times in his or her treatment.

## VENIPUNCTURE/BLOOD DRAW

Venipuncture is the simple act of obtaining a blood sample from the patient's vein. This is one of the more familiar procedures, even to people who don't have a major medical condition. Usually, the person obtaining the blood sample (a phlebotomist, medical tech, nurse, or physician) will search for a vein before actually inserting a needle through the skin. Often this searching means using a tourniquet (typically a large rubber band-like strap that is wrapped around the arm or leg), and for many children, the tourniquet is the most uncomfortable part of the procedure. By using a tourniquet, the veins in that extremity become more prominent, making it easier to get a good blood flow to the needle. The medical provider selects the most promising vein, applies the tourniquet, wipes the area with alcohol or another cleaning agent to minimize bacterial contamination, and inserts the needle into the vein. The needles come in many different shapes and sizes.

A thin section of tubing may be connected directly to the needle that feeds the blood into a syringe, or the needle may be attached directly to the tubes that hold the blood for the lab. Once enough blood has been obtained, the provider releases the tourniquet and removes the needle.

Often, children are "hard sticks"; either their veins are too small or difficult to locate or they kick and scream so much that the needle misses its mark. These misses are less common in providers who are used to working with children, but even the most experienced phlebotomist can miss on a blood draw.

In some medical centers, a cream is applied to the skin where they anticipate the blood will be drawn. This cream can numb the skin and make the blood draw much less painful for the child. Using the "magic cream" can be especially helpful for elementary-aged children, who know that a needle can hurt them but are old enough to realize that the cream really works at making the skin numb, and this helps them relax when the procedure is done. One of the downsides to using this cream is that it often makes the veins temporarily smaller (a process known as vasoconstriction) and thus more difficult for the provider to locate when getting the blood sample, so the child may end up being stuck more than once.

Heat is another thing that often makes the veins easier to work with. In young children, the provider will place a heat pack in the area where he wants to get blood. This helps to temporarily expand the veins (a process known as vasodilation), giving the needle a slightly larger target for the blood draw. Some medical companies are combining heat with the cream that numbs the skin, hoping that this will give patients the best possible chance for a successful blood draw.

## IV PLACEMENT

An intravenous catheter, or IV, is a plastic cannula that is inserted into the vein over a needle introducer. By inserting the catheter directly into the blood stream, patients can have fluids and medicines given to them in a controlled setting. The process of placing an IV is very similar to venipuncture, with the exception of the needle being removed from the thin plastic tube before the IV is used. Often, if the IV is large enough, it can be used to get blood samples from the patient as well as for infusing medicines. Once it is in place, it gets heavily taped and secured so the child won't pull it out. Sometimes toddlers or infants have to have arm restraints (often called "No-No's") put in place to keep them from being able to pull at the IV. Most children, however, are fine after the IV actually gets taped down and even tend to forget that it's there.

Sometimes patients need more than one IV catheter to get all the medications they need. This is especially true for patients who are being cared for in an intensive care setting or who have just been diagnosed with their cancer illness. Most IVs need to be changed every 72 hours or so to help prevent inflammation of the veins (thrombophlebitis). Another problem with IV catheters is that they can infiltrate. This means that the IV gets displaced from its location in the vein and the medicine or fluids that are being given end up pooling in the subcutaneous tissue (soft tissue just under the skin), leading to swelling and discomfort.

## CENTRAL LINE PLACEMENT

*Jonathon hated needles. Every time he went to the doctor's office, he was worried that he would get a "shot." When he became sick from his cancer, he had to get a lot of blood draws to see what was going on with his body. He screamed and kicked every time someone tried to get a blood sample. We tried to work with him to explain what was going on, but he just got so worked up about everything that he couldn't relax. It got to the point where we had to have four people holding down this seven-year-old boy so he could get a test done. We were so happy when the central line was put in—finally, no more needles! [Excerpt from a conversation with a mother of a child with neuroblastoma.]*

A central line is essentially a large IV catheter that can be used for longer periods of time than a simple IV. Central lines are a big part of cancer therapy in modernized countries. They are not likely to infiltrate because the thin plastic tube is much longer than that used in a simple IV. There are temporary central lines, which are often placed by Pediatric Intensive Care Unit (PICU) staff, and more permanent central lines, which are typically placed in an operating room setting by a surgeon.

Central lines also have a nice feature of one, two, or three lumens (ports through which medications and fluids can be given), so the nurses can hook up one lumen to fluids and another to chemotherapy, antibiotics, or blood products at the same time. They are also usually very good for sending off blood specimens, keeping children from having to get stuck by needles at all hours of the day. When one of these lines is placed, the patient is usually asleep from sedating medications. The temporary lines are often inserted into one of the large veins in the neck, upper chest, or groin. The permanent lines are usually put into one of the large veins in the upper chest.

All of the central lines have potential complications. Blood clots sometimes form in the area of the line, and they are more likely to get contaminated by bacteria and other infections. However, when a child is getting many different types of medicines at the same time, the central line makes things easier for her. Another huge benefit to central lines in cancer therapy is related to chemotherapy infusions. Chemotherapy is often a caustic substance, and some medicines can cause significant tissue damage if they aren't given directly into the vein, which can sometimes occur with simple or peripheral IVs.

In the United States, almost every child with cancer who is expected to get any form of medical therapy will have a central line. There are two major types of permanent central lines: external lines (often called Broviacs or Hickmans, related to the company that makes them) and subcutaneous lines (often called Portacath or Mediport, again related to the manufacturer). Both of these types of lines are placed in the operating room and involve minor surgical procedures.

For the external lines, a small incision is made in the area under the collarbone. The surgeon feeds one end of the catheter into the superior vena cava (a large vein that leads directly to the heart), and then tunnels the other end of the catheter under the skin. The catheter then exits the skin through another small incision. The central line leaves the body as one tube (single-lumen), but in some cases it branches out into two (double-lumen) or three (triple-lumen) different ports. A sterile dressing is placed over the area where the line exits the skin to help prevent infections in that area. This dressing should be changed every few days, and this can be done at home or in the hospital.

The subcutaneous line is quite different from the external lines. It is completely under the skin and is usually located in the chest area in pediatric patients. The surgeon again makes a small incision in the upper chest and feeds the end of the catheter into the superior vena cava. The other end of the catheter is a small chamber called a port or portal. This port is placed into a pocket created by the surgeon between the muscle and the skin of the chest. You can actually see a lump under the skin, which is the port part of the central line. This area is where the nurses access the blood system. They use a special needle (a Huber needle) with a tube attached to it, and place the needle through the spot of skin directly over the port, going through the rubber top into the reservoir connected to the catheter. With children, the cream that numbs the skin is often used before the needle is inserted into the port. As time passes, children become more comfortable with the procedure, and their skin even gets insensitive to the needle, so they don't mind the needle stick.

There are pros and cons to both types of central lines, and many physicians have their personal preferences, often based on the age of the child and the type of cancer that needs to be treated. With the external lines, extra care has to be taken to keep the dressing dry, and often children are prevented from going swimming. External lines also have to be flushed every day to help prevent blood clots from forming inside the catheter. This can easily be done at home, but it adds one more job to the list for which parents are responsible when the child is out of the hospital. Treating institutions will instruct parents and other caregivers on how to care for these external lines.

These "permanent" central lines are usually removed within a few months of the end of the cancer treatment. The removal is typically done in the operating room or some other controlled setting. Occasionally they have to be replaced during the therapy. Sometimes they get colonized with bacteria (bacteria are living inside the line, causing the child to have repeated blood infections). Other times the lines may break, or they don't infuse appropriately and need to be changed. In many instances, though, the first central line that is placed for treatment is the only IV access that the patient needs for his entire course of therapy.

## PICC LINES

Peripherally Inserted Central Catheters, or PICC lines, are another type of central line used under certain circumstances. When a child first gets diagnosed with cancer, sometimes it is difficult to get one of the more permanent central lines placed in the first few weeks, and the treating physicians will place a PICC line instead. This line looks a lot like the simple IV. It is often placed in the bend of the arm like a regular IV, but the catheter is much longer and travels all the way up the arm into the larger blood vessels in the chest. These lines are usually put in while the child is asleep from sedating medications.

PICC lines are good because they give a greater degree of certainty that the medicines are going into the vein than does a simple IV. In older children, the lines are large enough that blood can easily be drawn off the PICC line for routine blood tests as well. However, in younger children, the lines are often too small to be able to get a good blood return, so it's necessary that these children get needle sticks for their labs. Also, PICC lines are not meant to stay in place for prolonged periods of time, so most childhood cancer patients with PICC lines will eventually go on to have a permanent central line placed.

## LUMBAR PUNCTURE

*With Kayla's leukemia, we got pretty used to her having spinal taps done. The worst part was that she couldn't have anything to eat or drink before the procedure because of the sedation medicines that the doctors used. She would come to the clinic in the morning, and the nurses would put some cream on her back to make the area numb. Then the doctor would examine her and talk to us about the procedure. Once the medicines were ready, we would go to a special "procedure" room, where she was able to watch TV or listen to music. The nurses would put stickers on her chest and finger to keep track of her heart rate, and they would put a blood pressure cuff on her arm or leg. Then the doctors would give her the medicine to make her sleepy. Sometimes she fought the medicines, but most of the time she just looked at me funny and said things like "You have two heads," or "Why are you blue?"*

*After she was "feeling no pain," the doctors would put a needle into her lower back and collect the spinal fluid. Then they would give her the yellow chemotherapy medicine. Once the chemotherapy treatment was done, we worked on getting Kayla awake and drinking. It usually took her about 15 or 30 minutes to wake up from the medicines. Most of the time, she didn't remember anything that they did to her. [Excerpt from a conversation with a mother of a child with leukemia.]*

A lumbar puncture, or spinal tap, may be required at the diagnosis of cancer and at various times during treatment. In most instances, the procedure is done using some form of sedation to keep the child comfortable. The doctor or nurses may put some lidocaine cream on the skin over the area where the procedure will be done, or xylocaine may be injected directly into the skin at the same location. The child is usually placed on her side, with her knees pulled up and her chin pulled down towards the chest. Occasionally, older children or teenagers are allowed to sit up with their backs curved outward. This helps open up the spaces in between the bones of the spine (vertebral bodies), which often makes the procedure more successful. The doctor usually locates a space that is in line with the top of the hip bones (iliac crests), and after the area has been cleaned, the provider inserts a spinal needle into the space around the spinal cord that contains cerebrospinal fluid, or CSF.

CSF is a clear, almost water-like fluid that bathes the brain and spinal cord. A sample of the fluid is placed in a small plastic tube, taken to the lab, and processed to look for cancer cells that may be hiding around the brain or spinal cord. This fluid actually drips out of the needle, and it sometimes takes several minutes for enough fluid to be collected. Occasionally, the CSF is difficult to obtain, and sometimes a bloody sample is all that drips out of the needle. While it isn't an ideal sample, it can still have some value to the treating providers. In some diseases like leukemia, after the fluid is collected, the doctor will infuse chemotherapy (through the same needle that was used to obtain the fluid sample) into the space to mix with the CSF, helping to kill any tumor cells that may be present.

One of the biggest parental concerns about this procedure is that the spinal needle may damage the spinal cord. Fortunately, this risk is minimal because of the anatomy of the spinal cord within the spine. The bulky spinal cord is a thick, almost rope-like structure that comes from the base of the brain. This thick area of the spinal cord usually ends in the upper lumbar spine region, and only single separate nerves are present in the area where the procedure is typically done. With these nerves floating in the spinal fluid, it makes it very difficult for a needle to actually touch or damage one of these separate nerves. As with any procedure that involves a needle, other risks include bleeding and infection. The procedure is done in a sterile fashion, meaning that the area is prepared with cleansing solution, draped with sterile drapes, and the physician wears sterile gloves when doing the lumbar puncture.

With the exception of leukemia and some brain tumors, this procedure may be a one-time test. Most leukemia patients will have the procedure performed several times during the course of their treatment, almost always with concurrent chemotherapy infusion into the CSF, otherwise called intrathecal chemotherapy infusion. The results of the test are usually available within a few hours to a couple of days.

## BONE MARROW ASPIRATE

*There were so many tests done when Joel was diagnosed with neuroblastoma, but the one I hated the most was the bone marrow test. It just seemed so brutal to be pushing a needle into someone's hip like that. I was so happy that he was able to sleep during the procedure—it was much harder for me to watch the test than for him to actually have the test done. He never remembered anything about it except that his backside was pretty sore for a couple of days. [Excerpt from a conversation with a mother of a child with neuroblastoma.]*

A bone marrow aspirate is another test performed in the evaluation of many different types of cancers. This test is done to look for cancer cells that are deposited in the bone marrow. All leukemia patients by the definition of the disease have cancer cells in the bone marrow, so this test is extremely important to monitor the progress of therapy in these patients. Some solid tumors can also metastasize to the bone marrow, and this can have important prognostic significance for the child.

Bone marrow procedures are often done after the child has been given some form of sedation medication to make him more comfortable. The child can be placed in different positions, depending on which bone will be used for the procedure. Most commonly, the sample is taken from the posterior iliac crest, which is an area of the hip bone at the top of the buttocks, a couple of inches from the spine. Sometimes, in larger patients, it can be difficult to feel this part of the hip bone, so the sample is taken from the anterior iliac crest, which is the part of the hip bone that you can feel from the front. In infants, it can be hard to get an adequate sample from these areas, so sometimes the tibia (shin bone) is used.

In all locations, the procedure usually involves numbing the skin with either lidocaine cream or xylocaine injections. The area is cleaned, and a special bone marrow aspirate needle, which contains a stylet, is inserted into the bone. Once it is securely in the bone, the stylet is removed, and a syringe is attached to the aspirate needle. The amount of specimen needed varies according to the tests that need to be run, but usually several milliliters (one to three teaspoons) of liquid bone marrow are removed. The bone marrow, which looks almost exactly like blood, may be directly placed on microscope slides, or it may be put in tubes for later analysis. A good bone marrow aspirate specimen contains spicules (very small dust-like pieces of bone). If the aspirate does not contain spicules, the doctor may decide to reposition the needle or repeat the test.

In patients who have been diagnosed with leukemia, the normal bone marrow has been replaced by abnormal leukemia cells. This can make the procedure more difficult, and sometimes multiple attempts may be necessary.

After the sample has been obtained, the needle is removed and a pressure bandage is applied to the area. The most common side effects of the procedure are infection and bleeding, but the area is cleaned, prepped, and draped in a sterile fashion, and the pressure bandage helps to keep post-procedure bleeding to a minimum.

## BONE MARROW BIOPSY

The bone marrow biopsy has many similarities to the bone marrow aspirate, and it is usually done in conjunction with the aspirate procedure. In this procedure, instead of trying to get a sample of liquid marrow, the provider is actually looking to obtain a small piece of solid bone. The bone is about as thick as a strand of spaghetti, and is usually one-half inch to one inch in length. The bone sample is helpful in giving a sense of the architecture of the bone; it helps in determining if there are too many or not enough cells in the bone marrow, and it is useful for picking up clumps of solid tumor cells that have metastasized to the bone marrow.

The location of the bone marrow biopsy parallels the site of the bone marrow aspirate. Sedation and preparation for the procedure are also the same.

The needle used in the biopsy is a little larger and is sometimes referred to as a Jamshidi needle. Sometimes the doctor needs to make a small incision in the skin to help the needle get through. The needle is inserted into the bone and anchored into place. The stylet is removed, and the hollow needle is pushed further into the bone to core out a small piece, much as an apple corer removes the center of an apple. The needle is then taken from the skin, hopefully keeping the core piece of bone inside the hollow section of the needle. The bone is then taken from the needle and prepped for processing. One of the most problematic parts of this procedure is having the piece of bone stay behind in the patient after the needle has been removed. Other risks include bleeding and infection, but the area is treated as in the bone marrow aspirate to minimize these risks.

Some worry that the missing piece of bone will cause long-term damage to the hip, but the piece is very small, and the bone will heal with time, even if the procedure has to be repeated at various points during the treatment. With the exception of small scars in the skin at the site of the procedure, usually there is no other long-term effect of the bone marrow procedures.

## ECHOCARDIOGRAM

An echocardiogram, or echo, is an ultrasound of the heart. Its major function is to assess the strength of the patient's heart. Some of the chemotherapy agents used in pediatric cancer therapy can affect the heart function, making it pump blood less efficiently. This procedure uses the same technology as a prenatal ultrasound; a transducer, or ultrasound probe, which transmits high-frequency sound waves, is placed on the chest and abdomen. The transducer is able to pick up the echoes of the sound waves and send them to the machine as electric impulses, which are then converted into images of the heart.

The transducer is coated with the same "goo" that is used in prenatal ultrasounds to help with the transmission of the images. It is painless for the child, but younger children may still be scared by the machine. For children who receive chemotherapy that can affect their heart function, this test will need to be repeated at regular intervals (in some cases yearly) after their treatments have ended for an indefinite period of time.

## ELECTROCARDIOGRAM

An electrocardiogram, or ECG/EKG, is a test that records the electrical activity of the heart. It is often done in conjunction with the echocardiogram to help give more complete information about the heart. While the echo can look at the size and pumping strength of the heart, the ECG gives information about the electrical conduction of the heart. It can detect arrhythmias (irregular or atypical beating patterns), heart blocks, electrolyte disturbances, and other medical problems that can affect the rhythm of the heart's beating.

Several leads are attached to the body in various places to help the machine get the proper electrical conduction. Stickers are placed in the correct positions, and then the wires that are hooked into the ECG machine are clipped to the stickers. Once the leads are properly attached, the machine "reads" the heart's activity for several seconds and prints the activity on a special piece of graph paper in the machine. The child must stay still during the procedure, which can be very difficult for younger children.

Procedures similar to ECGs may be done under certain settings in the hospital, especially when the patient is very sick. Patients who are hooked up to cardiorespiratory monitors have similar stickers in place with wires attached to the monitor to help the physicians keep an eye on the electrical activity of the heart.

## RADIOLOGY STUDIES

### X-rays

Rontgen, or X-rays, will be done in practically every child who has the diagnosis of cancer. Patients who have leukemia or lymphoma will have X-rays to check the placement of their central lines or to rule out enlargement of lymph nodes in the chest. Patients with bone tumors will have these "plain films" done to look at the changes in their bones, not only at diagnosis but after their treatment has begun. Chest X-rays can be used to detect pneumonia. An abdominal X-ray can tell if the intestines are blocked (ileus) or perforated, and can sometimes even pick up things like kidney stones or gallstones.

These studies are relatively simple to do; the patient has to be positioned appropriately to get pictures of the correct part of the body. The test is quick once the patient is in the right position, and there is no real discomfort with the procedure.

### Ultrasounds

An ultrasound, or sonogram, is most often used in pediatric cancer patients with tumors in their abdomen, such as Wilms' tumors or other kidney tumors. They may also be used in patients to check for blood clots in their arms or legs or to see if they have fluid in their lungs. Almost exactly like an echocardiogram, a transducer, or ultrasound probe, which transmits high-frequency sound waves, is placed over the area being examined. As in a prenatal ultrasound, the transducer is coated with a type of gel that helps in transmitting the sound waves to and from the area being examined.

Ultrasounds are non-invasive and they do not expose the patient to any radiation. They typically are painless and cause minimal to no anxiety for the patient getting the test. One of their downsides is the lack of detail provided by the sound wave images. Often, if the results of the ultrasound are inconclusive, the provider will go on to order a more detailed examination, such as a CT scan or an MRI.

## CT Scans

Computed tomography, otherwise known as CT or "Cat" scans, are able to give physicians much more detailed images than regular X-rays, and the procedure takes less time than an MRI. The downsides to CT scans are the amount of radiation that the patient is exposed to and the contrast that is usually given to get the best picture.

The patient lies on a stiff, straight table that can be raised and lowered as needed. The table is then fed into a doughnut-shaped machine, where the images are taken. A red laser light helps the radiology technician align the child appropriately in the scanner. Once the patient is in place, the machine whirs into action, taking pictures as the coils rotate around. The entire body can be scanned in a couple of minutes.

There are two general types of contrast—oral and intravenous. Oral contrast is used primarily in scans involving the abdomen or the pelvis. This contrast is given to give the radiologist a better view of the intestines, and it helps them differentiate intestines from lymph nodes and other vital organs. There are several different "flavors" of the barium contrast available, and the patient drinks the chilled barium over a period of a couple of hours before the pictures are taken. It can be very difficult to get children to drink this material, and in the youngest patients, occasionally it has to be given through a tube that travels through the nose, down the esophagus, and into the stomach (nasogastric tube). Sometimes oral contrast is not needed, but in most situations it is preferred.

Intravenous contrast is given through a peripheral IV line during the scan. After some of the pictures have been taken, someone in the radiology department has the contrast infused through the IV (often given by a machine). This contrast is usually iodine-based and can cause some significant reactions. Almost everyone has some sensation from the contrast. As the contrast goes into the IV and spreads throughout the body, it is accompanied by a strange warm sensation. Sometimes the lips may start to tingle as well. The warmth spreads from the face downward. Occasionally, the contrast makes the patient have the false sensation that they have urinated during the scans.

## MRI Scans

*The MRI tests were quite an experience. I would sit in the room while Veronica had the test done, and it was SO loud. I don't see how she could stand being in that small tube, staying so very still while that machine kept making clanging and banging noises. There was a rhythm to the sounds that were made, and I guess that the sounds had something to do with the type of pictures being taken, but it was really strange. [Excerpt from a conversation with a mother of a child with osteosarcoma.]*

Magnetic resonance imaging, or MRI, is a type of scan best suited for examining muscle, bone, or brain tumors. MRI gives a very detailed image without exposing the patient to potentially harmful radiation. Unfortunately, it takes much longer than a CT scan, it is associated with a lot of loud noises that can scare children, and it can make many people feel claustrophobic.

Because the major component of the MRI machine is a magnet, patients are forbidden to bring any type of metal into the MRI room. Also, if patients have metal implanted into their body for some reason, they may not be able to have an MRI. All of these things are discussed prior to the scan being done.

The patient has to remain very still for this procedure, and since it is a lengthy procedure, many younger children require sedation. Others who are nervous in tight spaces may need some sort of anxiolytic (anti-anxiety medicine) to help them tolerate being cooped in the small space for such a long time.

The MRI is less suited for imaging areas that don't remain still, such as the lung and intestines. There are specific cardiac MRIs that can be done in the right setting for the right patient. The MRI is most commonly used for following solid tumors in the bones, brain, or muscles.

As in CT scans, IV contrast is often used to help make the different types of tissues easier to see. In tumors, IV gadolinium contrast is very important to determine if the area has "contrast enhancement." This enhancement, or prominence of the area with scanning, can help radiologists narrow down which type of tumor is present. Like the contrast given during CT scans, the MRI IV contrast can also cause some interesting sensations in patients receiving the infusion.

# NUCLEAR MEDICINE STUDIES

## PET Scan

A PET (positron emission tomography) scan is one of the relatively newer scans used in pediatric cancer monitoring. It gives a three-dimensional image of the patient, and areas of concern (like tumors) "light up" on the scan. The PET scan is useful because it is able to image the entire body without exposing the patient to significant amounts of radiation. Unfortunately, like the MRI, the scan itself can take a few hours to complete, so it may require sedative medications in younger children. When a child is sedated, they may need to have a urinary catheter placed to keep them from contaminating their clothing or the scan table from radioactive urine, thus complicating the radiologist's interpretation of the images that are taken.

The patient is not allowed to eat anything for a few hours before the scan and should not be taking any sort of steroid medication (unless required for their chemotherapy treatment) when the scan is done because this can affect the glucose levels in the body.

After an IV is placed, an injection of a radioactive substance attached to a natural body compound (usually a form of glucose) is given to the patient. Cancer cells in general grow rapidly and need nutrition to grow, so they are likely to have a significant accumulation of this radioactive glucose, which allows the cells to be seen by the PET scan machine. It takes around 30 to 90 minutes for the substance from the injection to travel through the body and collect in the cancerous cells. While waiting for this to happen, it is important for the child to remain fairly still because use of the muscles will increase their glucose uptake and keep the special radio-labeled glucose from going to the cancerous cells.

The patient lies down on a table attached to a machine that looks like a large doughnut, similar to the CT scanner. Once the child is in position, the scanning takes 30 minutes to an hour.

PET scans are sometimes done in machines called "PET-CT scanners." These machines offer the advantage of getting a CT image at the same time as the PET scan image, which helps the radiologist correlate findings on one scan type with findings on the other. PET images were once used only in pediatric lymphoma patients, but now they are used in many other solid tumors as well.

## Bone Scan

A bone scan is similar to the PET scan in that a radioactive substance is injected into the body through an IV and collects in the bones, specifically in areas of the bone that have a lot of activity or change. Some types of tumors will metastasize to the bones, leading to broken down areas of the bone, which are more likely to take up more of the radioactive tracer. The bone scan will not detect tumor cells in parts of the body other than the bones, so it is not a useful tool for many patients.

As in a PET scan, it takes time for the tracer to travel throughout the body, perhaps as long as four hours, before the pictures can be taken. Once the tracer has deposited in the bones, the patient is placed on a table so the technicians can start the special camera that is designed to pick up radioactivity. Similar to the PET scan, the bone scan looks at the entire skeleton. The scan itself takes up to an hour, so there are instances where smaller children will need sedation medication.

## MIBG

An MIBG scan, or metaiodobenzylguanidine scan, is used in a special group of tumors called neuroendocrine tumors. The most common neuroendocrine tumor seen in pediatric patients is neuroblastoma. Children with neuroblastoma will have this test many times during the course of their treatment and often for several years after the treatment has finished.

MIBG is a substance similar to adrenaline, which is labeled with a radioactive tracer. The labeled MIBG is injected through an IV and allowed to go through the blood stream to areas in the body that accumulate this substance, specifically tumors that have a high affinity for MIBG, such as neuroblastoma.

Before having an MIBG scan, the patient will need to do some prep work. Specifically, he needs to take iodine for a short period of time before the injection and for several days after the injection. This is meant to protect the thyroid gland from any radioactivity related to the MIBG injection, since the thyroid gland is so sensitive to radiation and also has an affinity for MIBG.

In an MIBG scan, the patient has to have pictures taken over a period of a few days. The MIBG tracer takes longer to accumulate in the tumor tissues than a PET scan or bone scan, so in some instances it can take 72 hours or more. It is not uncommon for a child to have pictures taken 24, 48, and 72 hours after the injection has been given, so a little more planning is required when getting this test scheduled.

## SURGICAL PROCEDURES

Many different types of surgical procedures may be performed in cancer patients, and naturally the type and location of the cancer helps determine what type of surgery will be performed. Some of the more commonly encountered surgical specialties include pediatric surgery, neurosurgery, orthopedic oncology, and urology.

The degree of preparation for the surgery depends on the type of surgery being performed. Almost all patients preparing for surgery will have to spend some time refraining from eating or drinking so they can be ready to receive the anesthetics provided to put them to sleep. Anesthesiologists want people to have an empty stomach when they are given these medicines to help keep them from aspirating (inhaling) any of the stomach contents when they are anesthetized. The patient will often have to refrain from eating or drinking anything from the night before until the time of the procedure.

On arrival at the surgical suite, the patient will be dressed in the appropriate hospital attire, and many different doctors, nurses, and technicians will meet the patient and her family to discuss the planned procedure, its potential complications, and the care during and after the surgery. If the child does not already have some sort of IV access, an IV will be started for hydration therapy. Often, the providers will give the patient some special "cocktail" of medicines to help her forget or at least be less worried about her immediate surroundings. In pediatric medicine, usually the parents are encouraged to stay with the child until she is actually taken back into the operating room. After the child is taken to the operating room, the parents and family members are asked to wait close by in specific locations for updates from the surgical team.

Once the child is taken back to the operating room, they will be placed on the operating table and prepared for the surgical procedure. The anesthesiologist will start medications to help the patient be completely unaware of his surroundings and will usually intubate the patient by inserting a plastic breathing tube into his trachea while delivering air through this tube into the patient's lungs. All of this is done in a closely monitored setting, where the heart rate and oxygen levels of the child are watched to ensure that he is getting enough air or oxygen in his system.

Once the patient is completely sedated and the anesthesiologist is in control of the breathing, the surgeon will prepare the area being operated on. This usually means cleaning the area and covering the rest of the patient in sterile drapes. The type of surgery being performed will determine the type of incision the surgeon makes. Some procedures are done with video cameras and others are done in a more "open" manner.

If a video-assisted surgical procedure is to be done, the surgeon usually makes several small incisions in various locations to give the best view of the area inside the patient. Video-assisted procedures in general have smaller incisions, and therefore less recovery time. However, in some circumstances, the surgeon is unable to actually get a good enough view of the area in question with the video equipment, so the procedure may be changed to an open surgical procedure.

Open surgical procedures involve longer incisions, but they also give the surgeon more room to work. Often when a surgeon is looking to remove a significant cancerous growth, the open procedure is preferred, because it allows the surgeon to see if there has been any spread of the cancer to other parts of the body. Unfortunately, the open procedures are more likely to leave large scars and require a longer recovery time in general.

For certain types of surgeries it is critical to have the right type of qualified specialist to do the procedure. One example is a patient with an undiagnosed bone tumor that needs to be biopsied. When a bone tumor is biopsied, the route that the surgeon takes to get the piece of tissue can have an important role in preventing the spread of the tumor to the surrounding area. Some surgeons might not take the correct approach when doing the biopsy, and this could be harmful for the child in the long run.

Once the child has finished her surgical procedure, the anesthesiologist will allow her to wake up. In most instances, once the child is ready, the tube will be removed from her airway, allowing her to breathe on her own once again. In some circumstances, the plan will be to keep the child on the ventilator (breathing machine) for a while after the surgery to allow more time to recover from the procedure. The patient will spend time recovering in the PACU (Post-Anesthesia Care Unit). The amount of time required in the PACU depends on how well the child is doing after surgery. Often the parents can visit with the child at this time, providing the child comfort as she awakens from the anesthetics.

After the PACU time is complete, the child may be allowed to go home, or he may be kept in a hospital room, depending on how involved the surgery was and the expected recovery time. Common post-operative complications include fevers and nausea or vomiting. Fevers often happen after surgery because the patient doesn't take deep enough breaths to keep the lungs open and free from something called atelectasis. The fever is not usually related to an infection if it happens only once or twice during the 24 hours or so after the surgery. Any nausea and vomiting is usually related to the anesthetic, and patients can be treated for this with special medicines, either at home or in the hospital setting.

# Chapter 9

## CHEMOTHERAPY AND TAKING MEDICINES

Chemotherapy is the term used for medicine given to fight cancerous cells. Most chemotherapy works by attacking cells that are dividing rapidly. Cancer cells in general, and especially childhood cancer cells, tend to fit that description; they grow and divide quickly. There are, however, other cells in the body, normal cells, that also fit that description. Cells in the gastrointestinal tract, such as those lining the inside of the mouth and the intestines, are rapidly dividing cells. Hair growth is a relatively rapid process. Blood cells also have a rapid growth cycle. Keeping this basic idea about chemotherapy in mind can help one conceptualize the reasons behind many of the side effects of these medications.

The idea of "chemotherapy" was first conceived in the 1940s with nitrogen mustard, which was initially used as a chemical warfare agent. Autopsies of people who had been exposed to this agent led scientists to think that it could be used as an anti-cancer therapy, and it showed some initial success in patients with lymphoma.

Another discovery was made when it was noted that folic acid (a vitamin that has a prominent role in DNA metabolism) actually seemed to make leukemia cells grow. Scientists took this concept and developed medications (called antifolates) that were antagonistic to folic acid. These medicines were then found to be effective in inducing a remission of ALL in children.

Some chemotherapy agents are actually derived from common plants. Vincristine is an agent in the group called vinca alkaloids that was created from the Madagascar periwinkle, or *Vinca rosea*.

When chemotherapy was first used in treating cancer, the agents were used by themselves, and when used alone, most of these agents were successful for only short periods of time. In the mid-1960s, multiple chemotherapy agents administered at the same time was tried for the first time. This plan followed the reasoning for treating tuberculosis. The bacterium responsible for the infection in tuberculosis was able to develop resistance to any one type of antibiotic given by itself. To get around the issue of resistance, many different antibiotics were given, thus preventing the bacteria from escaping the killing effect of antibiotics. In a similar way, cancer cells developed resistance to most chemotherapy agents when they were given by themselves, but the medical community started having significant success against cancer when multiple chemotherapy agents were given together, circumventing the cancer cells' way of surviving.

Another major concept in cancer chemotherapy is that of adjuvant therapy. In adjuvant therapy, chemotherapy is given not to cure the cancer, but as a means to make a different cancer treatment more effective. For example, with osteosarcoma, in most cases surgical resection alone is not enough to give a cure. Chemotherapy is given following the surgery as an adjuvant therapy, to support what the surgery was attempting to accomplish—to ensure that any remaining cancer cells are killed and not allowed to divide and grow further.

One of the major problems with chemotherapy is that most of the agents are in truth poisons. These agents work to kill the cancer cells in many instances, but their overall effectiveness is often limited by their side effects. Much of modern day oncology is working to maximize the effectiveness of these agents while minimizing their side effects. Some chemotherapy medicines are not effective in certain types of cancers, so more "toxic" combinations are required to get the same success. Some people are more sensitive to the side effects than others and cannot tolerate the "standard" doses of chemotherapy, thus limiting the potential effect of the chemotherapy on the cancer.

These agents are dosed based on the patient's body surface area, which is a calculated number determined by the patient's height and weight. In patients that are extremely overweight or in patients that are underweight due to their immediate illness, calculations may be based on the patient's "ideal" body surface area, using their height and a normal weight for their size.

# WORKING WITH CHILDREN TO TAKE MEDICINE

It can be extremely difficult to get a young child to take medicine. Some are blessed with children who love to take medicine, but most parents face a struggle when getting their child to take any type of medicine, from vitamins to antibiotics. Add to this the stress of taking a medicine such as "chemotherapy" that may taste pretty bad, and parents' days become even harder.

In terms of medication difficulties, leukemia medication is one of the toughest for parents. For ALL in particular, children are put on oral medicines from the very beginning and have to take some type of pill or liquid for the majority of the two to three years of treatment. They start their therapy with steroids (one of the worst tasting medicines ever). Children have to take this medicine two or three times a day for a month. Many parents go through various brands, different flavors, liquids, pills, dissolvable tablets, trying to find the magic formula that works best for them. There have been some newer formulations available that seem to taste a little better, but children still tend to resist this medicine in particular.

The most important thing to remember about getting children to take medicine is consistency. Parents need to make the child realize that he has no choice, that the medicine is a requirement, and there is no way that the child will get away with not taking it. When this approach is used, most children stop fighting the process within a matter of days because they know they can't win. However, if a parent gives in to the child's desires just one time, he will have hope that if he fights hard enough, the parent might give in again.

Parents usually become quite skilled in cutting or crushing tablets for their children. Many children learn to swallow pills at an early age to avoid some of the bad tastes in the liquid forms. Caregivers also get creative in ways to give the medicine. Some of the techniques for getting children to take their medicine are:

Mixing the liquid medicines with flavors available at many of the major pharmacy chains. Some patients prefer one flavor over another.

Using chocolate syrup to hide the bitter taste of some of the medicines.

Crushing tablets and putting them in cake icing to mask their taste.

Placing small tablets inside spoonfuls of gelatin dessert or ice cream to help them "slide down."

Softening a type of fruit candy chew in the microwave and wrapping it around the pill to make it more palatable.

"Training" children to take pills by having them swallow small candies without chewing. Once they have mastered this, they may be ready to move on to actual medications.

Most parents seem to prefer the pill forms of the medications in the long run, because they lead to less mess and less concern about the child getting only part of the dose. Some patients will spit out liquid medicines or drool out part of the dose as the medicine is being delivered. Other patient caregivers may have other tricks to help children take their medications. Many just experiment with different methods until they find one that works for their child.

## NAUSEA AND VOMITING WITH CHEMOTHERAPY

When you mention the word "chemotherapy" to someone, usually that person envisions medicines that make you lose your hair and make you throw up. While there is no way to prevent hair loss with some of these agents, there are many different ways to deal with the nausea and vomiting. Newer anti-nausea medicines have become available in the last few years, and what used to be a devastating side effect can now be managed relatively well for the majority of patients.

Physicians know ahead of time which chemotherapy agents are more likely to cause problems with nausea. It is important to remember that not all chemotherapy will cause nausea. The doctor will come up with an anti-nausea regimen based on the type of chemotherapy agents being given, the history of the child, and the way that the child handles the various anti-nausea treatments.

The majority of anti-nausea therapies used in pediatric oncology are medications. These medicines come in various forms—pills, liquid, dissolvable tablets, and intravenous doses. The doctor will likely give the IV forms to patients who are getting tougher regimens that require a stay in the hospital, while outpatient treatment for nausea will be handled with oral medications. There is an area in the brain known as the chemoreceptor trigger zone, which receives input from various medications to trigger nausea or vomiting. Newer generation anti-nausea medications, such as ondansetron and granisetron, work directly against neurotransmitter receptors in this chemoreceptor trigger zone, blocking the interaction of the chemotherapy with the receptors in this part of the brain.

Other anti-nausea medications include steroids, lorazepam, and metoclopramide. Some physicians will actually use a medical form of marijuana in certain circumstances to help treat chemotherapy-related nausea and vomiting. It is important to work with the doctors to *prevent* the nausea and vomiting from happening, because once a patient starts to get sick it can be very difficult to stop the cycle.

Some patients actually experience a syndrome where they may start to vomit if they just see certain things that they relate to their treatments. Children may become nauseated when they drive past the hospital or when they see certain people that they associate with their treatments. These feelings are real and can be very difficult to treat when they occur.

Other things that can help with chemotherapy-related nausea include encouraging the child to drink a lot of fluids, eating small amounts of only the things that really appeal to the child, avoiding certain smells, and distraction techniques. Some pediatric oncologists are investigating the use of acupuncture to help with nausea and vomiting in children as well.

## SPECIFIC CHEMOTHERAPY AGENTS

The following section will talk about individual chemotherapy agents, their major side effects, and major cancer uses.

### Methotrexate

Methotrexate is an antimetabolite, or antifolate, as mentioned above. It works by inhibiting folic acid metabolism, so when children are getting this medication, they should avoid most multivitamins, almost all of which contain folic acid. Methotrexate is not just for cancer therapy. It is also used in the treatment of many autoimmune illnesses (such as rheumatoid arthritis) and bowel disorders (such as Crohn's disease). It has also been used in the treatment of ectopic pregnancies (pregnancies where the fetus has implanted in a part of the body other than the uterus).

Methotrexate is a yellow colored medicine, and it can be given in many different forms. It can be given through the IV in small doses, large doses, or long (24-hour) infusions. In some instances it is given through an intramuscular injection. In others it is given by mouth, and in leukemia patients, it is also given directly into the spinal fluid through an intrathecal approach.

When given in pill forms, patients often have to take many of these pills at once. The tablets come only in one size, so the larger the patient, the more tablets she has to take. The most common timing for getting methotrexate pills is weekly, but occasionally, patients will need slightly different dosing.

Sometimes, when a patient is getting a significant amount of methotrexate, this can put the patient's body at risk for serious toxic side effects. Since methotrexate works to deprive cells of folic acid (a B vitamin), it works on cancer cells and normal cells alike. Fortunately, the effects on the cancer cells seem to occur more quickly than on the body's normal cells, so the key is to replace the folic acid in the body at the right time—after the cancer cells have been killed but before the body feels any toxic effects. The replacement of the folic acid is called a rescue with another medicine called leucovorin. Leucovorin is the active form of folic acid, otherwise known as folinic acid, and when it is replaced in the body, it works very quickly to get to the cells it needs to reach in the body. Good hydration is another key to helping the body rid itself of methotrexate. Methotrexate is eliminated from the body in the urine, so aggressive fluid administration can help keep methotrexate damage to a minimum.

When a patient is being treated with the longer 24-hour infusions of methotrexate, the physicians monitor the body's methotrexate levels very closely and will not discharge the patient from the hospital before knowing that the levels are in a safe range. These long infusions almost always require the leucovorin rescue therapy. Leucovorin can be given in a pill format or by IV, and it is given on a scheduled basis until the methotrexate levels are in the safe range. Patients will also be given aggressive IV fluid hydration during their hospital stay. Hospitalizations for these higher doses of methotrexate usually last for a few days, depending on how quickly the patient clears the methotrexate from her system.

The most common side effects from methotrexate include mouth and other gastrointestinal tract sores (otherwise known as mucositis), nausea, vomiting, skin changes, anemia, and low white blood cell counts. Methotrexate will almost always cause a change in the patient's labs, specifically their liver enzymes. While this is not a sign of any significant long-term liver damage, the number changes do occur and are expected by the treating physicians.

Many of the pediatric cancers are treated by methotrexate. Acute lymphoblastic leukemia (ALL) uses methotrexate in many different forms during therapy. It is also used in most forms of the non-Hodgkin's lymphomas. Some solid tumors benefit from methotrexate as well, such as osteosarcoma, and some types of brain tumors.

### Mercaptopurine/Thioguanine (6-MP/6-TG)

Mercaptopurine, otherwise known as 6-MP, and thioguanine, otherwise known as 6-TG, are chemotherapy agents from a group of drugs known as antimetabolites. They actually resemble normal cell nutrients that cells need to grow, so when the cancer cells take up this "fake" nutrient, it hinders their growth. Mercaptopurine and thioguanine play a major role in the treatment of acute lymphoblastic leukemia (ALL). However, mercaptopurine in particular has other medical uses. Some people take this medicine to treat inflammatory bowel diseases such as Crohn's disease and ulcerative colitis, and others use it to treat autoimmune diseases such as lupus and rheumatoid arthritis.

Mercaptopurine and thioguanine are both yellow-colored tablets. At one time, mercaptopurine was used as an intravenous medication, but today its use is in tablet format only. Since many of the patients with leukemia are quite young, getting them to take tablets can at times be difficult. This medicine also has to be timed appropriately to avoid interactions with food products. Most people take the medicine in the late evening; it needs to be taken at least two hours after and one hour before food intake, so many patients take the medicine right before going to bed. The other reason to take the medicine before sleep is that it can sometimes make people feel nauseous, so sleeping through the nausea helps patients feel better. Most patients getting treatment for ALL are taking one of these medications for months at a time, so it is crucial to have a plan that makes any potential side effects bearable.

This medicine is dosed based on the patient's body surface area. Many children require half-tablet doses, while some require more than a full tablet, depending on their size. Some people metabolize or break down these medications differently than others. There are genetic tests that can be done that help the doctors determine who needs to have the doses adjusted based on their body's use of the medication. People who have the different metabolism of 6-MP and 6-TG are more likely to have side effects from full doses of treatment, so it can be very important to adjust their doses when necessary.

One of the most common side effects from these medicines is lower blood cell counts. When the white blood cell count is low, the child is more likely to develop a serious infection, and often the oncologists will have patients stop taking this medicine for brief periods of time while waiting for the white blood cell count to recover. Other effects noted from the medicines are changes in liver function and fatigue. Usually, the changes to the liver are temporary and not significant enough to change the medication. Very rarely, the liver has more permanent changes that can lead to serious long-term problems. The long-term problems seem to be related more to thioguanine usage than mercaptopurine, so most treatment plans currently in use limit the amount of thioguanine given to patients.

## Doxorubicin/Daunorubicin/Idarubicin/Mitoxantrone

Doxorubicin (otherwise known as Adriamycin), daunorubicin, idarubicin, and mitoxantrone belong to a class of chemotherapy agents known as anthracycline antibiotics. Daunorubicin was discovered first, and it is actually related to a bacterium called *Streptomyces*. Doxorubicin was discovered a few years later and is the most commonly used medication in this group. These agents work by stopping DNA replication (reproduction) within rapidly dividing cells. They are commonly used in many different types of cancer therapy in children and in adults.

These medicines are all given in intravenous form when treating pediatric patients. Doxorubicin, daunorubicin, and idarubicin are all red liquids, while mitoxantrone is dark blue. Most people remember these medications by their distinct color. The IV infusions typically take an hour or less, depending on the dose and the patient. As in other agents, they are dosed based on the body surface area of the patient, so younger children will receive much lower doses than older teenagers. In the United States, this medicine is typically given only through a central venous catheter because there is significant risk to the patient if it goes directly into the skin and not into the vein. If a patient is receiving this medicine in a small, regular IV, and the IV infiltrates (starts infusing outside of the vein into the soft tissue around the blood vessel), it can cause severe skin damage that at times requires skin grafting and plastic surgery care.

There are several different side effects that are common with anthracyclines, including lower blood counts (which make patients more susceptible to infection), nausea and vomiting, and hair loss (which typically occurs three weeks or so after the start of the therapy). There have also been rare instances (less than 1 percent) of these medicines being associated with a secondary leukemia (leukemia caused by effects of the medicines in a patient who did not have that type of cancer to begin with).

The most well-known and potentially life-threatening effect from this medicine is cardiotoxicity, or problems with heart function. The effects on heart function are well documented and were quite prevalent in the early years of this medicine. Physicians now know that there is a relationship between the total amount of anthracycline medicine given and the risk of developing heart problems. There are also studies being done to determine if genetics plays a role in patients developing the heart problems. Younger-aged patients and patients who also receive any amount of radiation treatment to the heart are at higher risk of heart problems. There are times that the heart effects are so severe that the heart fails and significant medical interventions become necessary for treatment. There is a medicine that has undergone investigation as a potential heart protector for patients getting these anthracyclines called dexrazoxane, and some physicians will recommend this medicine to patients in certain circumstances. To prevent some of these problems, patients have echocardiograms performed at regular intervals to ensure that their heart function has not changed.

Anthracycline therapy is used in many different types of pediatric cancers, including leukemia, Hodgkin's and non-Hodgkin's lymphomas, osteosarcoma, rhabdomyosarcoma, other soft tissue sarcomas, Ewing's sarcoma, liver tumors, Wilms' tumor, and neuroblastoma.

**Bleomycin**

Bleomycin is a chemotherapy agent that, like the anthracyclines, is also an antibiotic formed from a bacterium called *Streptomyces*. It works by causing the DNA strands in cancer cells to break and, therefore, to be unable to replicate (reproduce). It is used in some specific forms of cancer therapy in pediatric and adult patients, such as Hodgkin's lymphoma and certain types of germ cell tumors or testicular cancers.

This agent is usually given intravenously, but it can also be given directly into the muscle or under the skin. This clear water-like fluid is typically given over a period of minutes to an hour. It is dosed for patients based on their body surface area. Common side effects of bleomycin include fever, rash, and changes in skin coloration. It can also make people feel tired or weak and can alter their taste of certain types of food. Hair loss is uncommon with this medication, but it can occur, typically around three weeks after the start of the therapy.

The most concerning side effect of bleomycin is pulmonary fibrosis. This is a chronic lung disease in which the lungs are replaced by a sort of scar tissue, making them less able to expand and deflate as before. These effects are worsened in people who also receive radiation therapy to their lungs or who are smokers. Pediatric patients over the age of five years will have tests of their pulmonary function (lung breathing capacity) before receiving this medicine and at key points during and after treatment. These pulmonary function tests, or PFTs, are simple breathing tests in which a machine measures how quickly air moves through the lungs and how much air the lungs can hold. The patient breathes forcefully into and out of the machine under guidance of the technician performing the test. If the lung function is not as good as expected, the oncologist may adjust the doses of the bleomycin therapy as needed.

**Busulfan**

Busulfan is a chemotherapy agent grouped in a class known as alkylating agents. These agents attach themselves to specific parts of the cancer cell's

DNA and prevent the DNA strands from separating. Separation of the strands is necessary for the DNA and the cancer cells to reproduce. Busulfan's use in pediatric cancer is typically limited to bone marrow transplantation, where it is used as part of the preparative (or conditioning) chemotherapy regimen prior to the patient receiving the bone marrow transplant.

This agent comes in two forms—a white tablet that is taken by mouth and a clear liquid that is given intravenously. Since this agent is widely used in preparation for bone marrow transplants, it is intentionally given to produce the side effect of significantly lowered blood cell counts. These lower numbers of white blood cells in particular put the patient at risk for serious infection. Other side effects include changes in the skin, fatigue, pulmonary fibrosis (see bleomycin), and seizures. Often, physicians will give patients anti-seizure medications to prevent the seizures from occurring. When seizures do happen, they are related to the medication and stop after the Busulfan has worn off. As in therapy with bleomycin, patients with busulfan over the age of five years will be asked to do pulmonary function testing to assess their lung health.

### Vincristine/Vinblastine

Vincristine and vinblastine belong to a class of agents known as vinca alkaloids. These chemotherapy medicines were actually derived from the Madagascar periwinkle, or vinca plant. They were first approved for chemotherapy use in the United States in the 1960s. Vincristine in particular is used in many different pediatric cancer treatments, including leukemia, lymphomas, rhabdomyosarcoma, Ewing's sarcoma, other soft tissue sarcomas, and some brain tumors.

These clear fluid medicines are given only intravenously. The amount of medicine given is typically pretty small, and it is given by "IV push," meaning that the medicine is just pushed through the syringe into the IV line by hand over a matter of seconds to a minute or two. These agents can cause problems if the IV is not correctly placed in the vein, because if it infiltrates, or spreads into the soft tissue surrounding the blood vessel, it can cause significant skin damage, almost like a burn.

The majority of side effects with vincristine and vinblastine are related to their effects on the nerves in the body. Nearly all patients will lose their reflexes (the jerking motion that is experienced when the doctor taps on the knee or ankle). Most patients experience some loss of sensation in their hands and feet, making it more difficult for them to do things that require fine motor skills, such as writing, drawing, and buttoning clothes. Other patients experience pain from the changes in the nerves, typically in locations like the thighs or the jaw. This pain can usually be managed by specific pain medication.

In some children, their ability to walk changes dramatically with this medication because it alters the sensation in their feet, making it difficult for them to tell when their feet are in the right position on the floor. Others have nerve problems that affect their intestines, making it difficult for them to have bowel movements. Most patients experience some amount of constipation, and others get so severe that they have obstipation (they are unable to eliminate any amount of stool). These side effects are managed by altering the doses of the medications as needed. The nerve effects usually are not permanent. Patients will recover nerve function with time after the treatment is complete.

Other side effects to the vinca alkaloids include potential hair loss or hair thinning, fatigue, and changes in taste sensation. Vinblastine in particular is more likely to lower the blood cell counts, making patients more at risk for infections or anemia.

### Actinomycin-D

Actinomycin-D is one of a class of antibiotics that has uses against cancer cells. It was isolated from a class of bacterium called *Streptomyces*. Actinomycin-D is an older chemotherapy agent that binds to the cancer cells' DNA and prevents it from be copied (a process known as transcription). It is commonly used in certain pediatric tumors, such as Wilms' tumor and rhabdomyosarcoma.

This medicine is given only intravenously. It is a clear yellow liquid that can be given over a few minutes. Common side effects include nausea and vomiting, lower blood cell counts, hair loss (typically occurs three weeks after starting the treatment), and fatigue. An acne-like rash can also occur from actinomycin-D administration. One of the more serious side effects is something called veno-occlusive disease (VOD) of the liver, in which the liver becomes enlarged, the patient retains excess fluid, and the patient becomes yellow, or jaundiced, from high levels of bilirubin in their system. This is treated by restriction of fluid intake and is usually a temporary side effect, although some patients have more serious consequences.

### Cyclophosphamide/Ifosfamide

Cyclophosphamide (also known as Cytoxan) and ifosfamide are chemotherapy medications that belong to a class called nitrogen mustard alkylating agents. Cyclophosphamide is also used in other non-cancer illnesses such as lupus-related kidney disease (severe lupus nephritis). These agents are transformed to active medicines by the liver, and these medicines link to the cancer cells' DNA, causing them to die.

These medicines are clear fluids that are almost always given intravenously in pediatric cancer patients. The medicine itself is typically infused over an hour or so through the IV. However, the medicine often needs to be given with a significant amount of IV fluid hydration, and this hydration can take several hours (sometimes requiring the patient to stay overnight in the hospital). This aggressive IV fluid hydration is done to prevent one of the more serious side effects of these medicines—hemorrhagic cystitis. Hemorrhagic cystitis is an inflammation of the bladder that can lead to significant amounts of blood and blood clots in the urine. Hemorrhagic cystitis is not as common as it once was due to aggressive prevention measures such as IV fluids and MESNA. MESNA is an agent given to protect the bladder from the toxic effects of these medications. It binds to one of the active compounds formed in the liver (acrolein) and prevents this active product from causing significant bladder inflammation.

Other common side effects related to cyclophosphamide and ifosfamide include nausea and vomiting, mouth sores, hair loss (typically occurs three weeks after starting the therapy), fatigue, and lower blood counts (which put the patient at risk for serious infection). These medicines have also been associated with infertility (depending on the dose of the medication, sex of the patient, and age of the patient at the time of treatment) and the development of another type of cancer, such as leukemia or bladder cancer. While these risks are low, patients are monitored for these problems for years after their treatment has been completed.

Cyclophosphamide and ifosfamide have uses in many different types of pediatric cancers, including acute lymphoblastic leukemia, lymphomas, osteosarcoma, rhabdomyosarcoma, Ewing's sarcoma, other soft tissue sarcomas, neuroblastoma, and Wilms' tumor.

### Asparaginase

Asparaginase (L-asparaginase) is a chemotherapy agent that works on depriving cancer cells of an amino acid (protein building block) called asparagine. There are several different forms of asparaginase used in pediatric patients. Older forms include E. coli asaparagniase (based on the *Escherichia coli* bacterium), and Erwinia asparaginase (based on the *Erwinia* bacterium). The form most commonly used today is PEG-asparaginase (pegylated asparaginase), where a molecule called polyethylene glycol is attached to asaparaginase, making it more stable and longer lasting.

All forms of asparaginase are typically given as an intramuscular injection and are used almost exclusively in acute lymphoblastic leukemia (ALL) patients and some non-Hodgkin's lymphoma patients. The older forms of this clear liquid medication are given every couple of days for certain periods of time to keep high enough levels of the medication in the body. The newer PEG-asparaginase form can be given on one day and last for several weeks, thus eliminating some shots for pediatric patients, which is very important to most patients.

One of the most common side effects from this medicine is an allergic reaction, which can manifest as redness at the site of the injection, a more generalized rash, or more seriously, airway swelling and difficulty breathing. Some patients may be allergic to one form of the medication but have no problems with other forms, so often physicians will try different forms before eliminating this form of therapy. Other uncommon but potential side effects include pancreatitis (inflammation of the pancreas with symptoms of abdominal pain and difficulty eating) and changes to the blood's clotting (coagulation) system. This disregulation of the clotting system can cause patients to be more likely to bleed or more likely to develop blood clots, with the most serious events potentially leading to a stroke.

## Steroids/Prednisone/Decadron

Steroids are a common medication used by many patients for a variety of illnesses, including asthma, poison ivy reactions, allergies, lupus, and disorders of inflammation in the body. They are also a key component to leukemia and lymphoma therapy. They are not related to the steroids that athletes are known to take for muscular enhancement. The steroids most commonly used in pediatric cancer patients are prednisone and decadron. The way that these medicines work against cancer cells is not fully understood, but they are very potent agents used early in the diagnosis of certain pediatric cancers.

These steroids can be given in many different ways, including pills or liquid taken by mouth, clear fluid given through the IV, or shots given into the muscles. Most of the time, oncologists use the forms that the patient can take by mouth. Steroid doses used in the treatment of pediatric cancer are often higher than doses given for other illnesses, so the potential side effects can also be greater. The most common side effects include increased irritability and moodiness, increased appetite, increased blood pressure, increased blood sugar levels, increased weight gain, problems with sleep, and irritation to the stomach. Some of these side effects require other medical interventions for treatment, such as insulin for patients with extremely high blood sugar levels, and antacids for patients with stomach irritation. Some later effects noted in patients with long-term steroid use include cataracts and weakening of the bones (osteoporosis). Steroids also affect the body's immune system and make patients more susceptible to getting infections.

One other key problem with using steroids is related to the body's own natural steroid production. The body needs to produce steroids at certain times of stress to help give the body a natural boost. If you give a person extra steroids at significant doses for long periods of time, you suppress the body's normal steroid production and make it slow to respond to steroid needs at times of stress. It can take time for the body to recover, and sometimes the physicians will do tests to check the body's production of the steroid cortisol.

Another use for steroids in patients with cancer is to decrease swelling or inflammation. This is particularly important in some patients with brain tumors, where swelling can lead to serious life-threatening complications. The steroids used in this case are typically given through the IV at high doses at the beginning of the diagnosis and following any surgical procedures done to the brain tumor.

### Cisplatin/Carboplatin

Cisplatin (also known as cisplatinum) and carboplatin are platinum-based chemotherapy agents that also belong in the category known as alkylators. These agents get worked into the cancer cells' DNA and make it impossible for the DNA to duplicate. These agents are used in pediatric patients with certain types of sarcomas, carcinomas, brain tumors, and germ cell tumors.

Cisplatin and carboplatin are clear fluids that are given through the intravenous route. They are typically infused over an hour or two and are often accompanied by a significant amount of IV hydration. This is done to protect the kidneys from side effects from these medications. One of the more common side effects of cisplatin in particular is nephrotoxicity (kidney damage), and this can sometimes be prevented by aggressive fluid intake. Patients will have their kidney function monitored very closely during and after treatment. If the kidney function decreases significantly during treatment, the dosing of the cisplatin or carboplatin will be adjusted, and sometimes the treatments are eliminated altogether. Due to the effects on the kidneys, patients may waste certain electrolytes such as magnesium and potassium in their urine, so they may need to take electrolyte supplements.

These medications are some of the worst for causing patients to have nausea and vomiting, so aggressive anti-nausea medications are given in conjunction with cisplatin and carboplatin. They are also associated with hearing loss (cisplatin more so than carboplatin), and some patients require hearing aids after completing their treatment. Other side effects may include infertility, numbness or tingling in the hands or feet, hair loss, lower blood counts, fatigue, and changes in taste sensations.

## Etoposide

Etoposide, or VP-16, is a chemotherapy agent in the class of epipodophyllotoxins, which is derived from a toxin found in the mandrake root. These agents work against an enzyme that works in the process of DNA replication (reproduction) and transcription, thus keeping cancer cells from dividing and reproducing. It is given in many different types of pediatric cancers, including leukemia, lymphoma (both Hodgkin's and non-Hodgkin's lymphomas), Ewing's sarcoma, germ cell tumors, and some brain tumors.

This clear fluid is usually given through the IV, but some patients are treated with pills, which are pale pink in color. It is usually given via IV over 30 to 60 minutes. Some patients have reactions to the infusion, such as low blood pressure or other allergic reactions such as a rash or difficulty breathing. The slower infusion rates are done to prevent some of these reactions from occurring.

Common side effects related to etoposide include lower blood cell counts, which make the patient more likely to develop serious infections, changes in taste sensations, nausea and vomiting, hair loss (typically occurs three weeks after the start of the treatment), and fatigue. It was previously discovered that higher total doses of this medicine make patients more likely to develop secondary cancers (cancers that are different than the one that they are receiving treatment for). The most common form of secondary cancer is acute myelocytic leukemia (AML), or an AML-precursor known as myelodysplastic syndrome. Physicians are careful to limit the total amount of this medicine given to patients, and this incidence has decreased in recent years.

# Chapter 10

# RADIATION THERAPY

When many people think of cancer treatments, one of their first thoughts is radiation therapy. Many adult patients with cancers like breast or lung cancer undergo various radiation treatments. Some people hear the term "radiation" and think of people in special suits with Geiger counters checking for radiation levels in the air following a radiation leak. Radiation is both a treatment for and a cause of cancer, and if not administered appropriately, it can do more harm than good.

The field of Radiation Oncology is quite complicated. Radiation therapy has evolved significantly in the past decades, and there are many different types of radiotherapy available today that were unheard of in the recent past. Some patients receive radiation to local sites of cancer disease, while others have their entire bodies irradiated in preparation for a bone marrow transplant. Knowing how much radiation to give in the correct doses at the correct time can be difficult, but great strides are being made in Radiation Oncology each year.

In pediatric and adolescent patients, radiation is usually given with the intent to cure the patient of his cancer. In adults, radiation is given also to cure, but it may, in addition, have the goal of relieving symptoms of the cancer. This is known as palliative treatment. Radiotherapy is most effective in treating tumors that have a rapid growth cycle, because these rapidly dividing cells are more likely to be destroyed by the radiation than more slowly evolving cells. The timing of the radiation also can be important in these cases, because some tumors are more likely to grow faster when they become small in size. In these cases, radiation therapy might be given twice a day in smaller doses to be more effective in killing the tumor.

In general, adults are often better suited to receive radiation treatments, because they have finished growing. In children and adolescents, radiation at high enough doses will stop their growth in the areas that are irradiated. Another problem with radiation therapy is that it is not always possible to focus the radiation solely on the cancer; normal tissue gets exposed to the radiation as well, and this normal tissue can be significantly affected by the radiation. Some areas of the body, such as the lungs and the heart, can take only a certain amount of radiation before being severely damaged. A tumor requires a very high dose of radiation to kill the cancerous cells, but that same dose may also damage the normal tissue beyond repair; so since doses have to be limited, they are not as effective against the cancer as they might be.

Most of the time, pediatric patients who are being treated with radiation therapy are also being treated with some form of chemotherapy. There are some chemotherapy medications that should not be given at the same time as the radiation treatments because of significant unwanted side effects. Sometimes, radiation therapy is used in combination with a surgical procedure, and timing the radiation treatments appropriately can be vital in allowing post-surgical tissues to adequately heal.

Radiation is dosed in units called gray (Gy) or centigray (cGy). Many people have heard also the term "rads," and one rad is equal to one centigray. The amount of radiation given to the patient depends on the type of tumor and its location. Some tumors require 60 Gy of treatment, while others are given only 12 or 18 Gy. The higher the total amount of radiation, the greater the risk for the patient, so higher doses are used only in cases where absolutely necessary. Over time, radiation oncologists have learned that breaking the high doses up into many smaller doses is less risky for the patient and prevents some of the immediate and long-term effects of the radiation. For example, a person receiving 55 Gy of radiation will likely get those treatments five days a weeks for a period of six and a half weeks. The "fractionation" of the dose and the length of treatment depends on the type of tumor and the circumstances surrounding the treatment.

*The first visit with the radiation doctor was pretty easy. We just talked about the treatment that Robert would receive and discussed some of the side effects of the treatment. He also had a CT scan to help the doctor focus the radiation to the right area of his neck. The next visit, for the simulation, was a little scary. Robert was put in the position for his radiation treatments. Then, the technician started molding a mask to his face and neck to make sure that his head would be in the perfect position for each radiation treatment. By fitting this mask to his face, he wasn't able to move his neck around during the treatments. They also wrote on him with a permanent marker to help the radiation technicians know how to direct the beams.*

*Once everything was set up, he started his treatments. They would fit his mask in place, then get him positioned for the radiation. The radiation itself was pretty quick. He looked kind of silly when he was done because he had these boxes and x's on his face left by the mask. He felt nauseated some afternoons, so we gave him medicine to treat his nausea. Towards the end of the six weeks, Robert was pretty tired and needed to take naps most days. [Excerpt from a conversation with a mother of a patient with nasopharyngeal carcinoma.]*

When a person needs radiation therapy as part of his treatment, there are some steps that must be taken to prepare the patient. First, the patient will consult with the radiation oncologist, the physician who actually provides the therapy. During that initial visit, the radiation oncologist will discuss the treatment plan and anticipated side effects of the therapy. The radiation oncologist works with other specialists in the radiation oncology department, such as the radiation physicist and dosimetrist to determine the best doses and the best way to administer the treatments to the patient.

After the details of the treatment have been decided, a "simulation" will be scheduled. During this visit, the patient usually will have imaging studies such as CT scans to help localize the exact area needing the treatment. The patient also will visit the radiation treatment room and undergo a process whereby the staff positions the patient as she will actually be positioned while receiving the radiation, and they may make some marks on her body to demonstrate the precise sites for therapy. Sometimes these marks are actual tattoos that are permanent reminders of the treatment given. Patients who are receiving radiation of the head or neck are frequently put in a specially molded mask that keeps the head in the best position possible for the treatment. These masks often have a mesh pattern on the inside, which can leave a crisscross pattern on the face after the treatment has been given.

The simulation visit typically takes much longer than the actual radiation treatments. Once the patient starts receiving the radiation itself, the visits are typically only a few minutes each day, with most of that time being used for setup and patient positioning. In pediatrics, sometimes children cannot reliably stay still during the radiation treatments. It is critical to stay completely still so that the radiation goes to the correct spot. If there is concern about patient movement, sedation medications will be given to the child every day of the therapy to help ensure their safety. Sedated visits take much longer than other routine visits, because the sedation medications take some time to begin working.

After receiving the radiation treatment, the child is permitted to go about his usual routine. There are typically no restrictions on where he can go or who he can see in terms of exposing someone to his irradiated body. The majority of radiation treatments given in children are not going to make them "radioactive" or a danger to others.

## HOW RADIATION THERAPY WORKS

The basic job of radiation therapy is to damage the DNA of the cells with which it comes in contact. The radiation beam works to ionize (change the numbers of protons and electrons) in the atoms that make up the DNA of the cancer cell. It also ionizes the water around the cells, forming free radicals (highly reactive electrons that can cause damage), which also damage the cancer cells. Cancer cells have more difficulty repairing the DNA damage than normal cells do, so they are more susceptible to being killed by radiation treatments.

There are several different types of radiotherapy being used in the United States. The most basic form of radiation therapy is called conventional external beam radiotherapy, which is a two-dimensional radiation delivery system. Single beams of radiation are given to the patient's cancer from different directions. This type of radiation must go through the normal tissue to get to the cancerous tissue, and it often goes a little past the tumor as well into even more normal tissue. In a growing child, this "scatter radiation" is often problematic and limits the dose of radiation that can be given to a certain area in the body.

Another form of radiotherapy is Three-Dimensional Conformal Radiotherapy, in which the beams are more easily conformed to the shape of the tumor, thus reducing the amount of radiation delivered to the normal surrounding tissues. In some patients, this allows the radiation oncologist to give a higher dose of treatment to the cancer, thus optimizing the chance of cure. A newer form of radiation that takes Three-Dimensional Conformal Radiotherapy a step further is Intensity-Modulated Radiation Therapy, or IMRT. This technique uses specific computing programs to control, or modulate, the intensity of the beam of radiation being delivered to the tumor. IMRT can conform better to unusually shaped tumors without exposing surrounding healthy tissues to as much radiation. IMRT is more complicated to plan than other radiation therapy, and special resources are often required. Both types of radiation therapies are dependent on the quality of the imaging used to identify the location of the tumor. If the scans that locate the tumor are unable to show all areas of disease, then the radiation treatment will miss important cancer cells that require the therapy.

One of the newest forms of radiation therapy having particular promise in pediatric patients is proton therapy. Unlike other forms of therapy that use electron beams, proton beams can stay very focused on the tumor tissue without spreading to the surrounding tissue. Protons have a specific range, and they will not penetrate beyond their range. Proton therapy is available only at specific centers in the United States and around the world. The equipment required for such treatment is extremely heavy and expensive, but the centers that provide this type of service have had good success.

Another form of radiation therapy is sealed source radiotherapy, or brachy-therapy. This type of therapy involves the implantation of a radioactive source inside or next to the tumor needing treatment. While this type of therapy is quite common in some adult cancers, such as prostate cancer, its use in pediatrics is limited.

## SIDE EFFECTS OF RADIATION THERAPY

Radiation therapy definitely has its share of potential side effects, with some occurring during treatment and some showing up much later after therapy is complete. The side effects depend on the location of the radiation, the amount of radiation given, and the surrounding normal tissues also affected. The side effects center on the fact that radiation therapy has to go through normal skin, muscle, soft tissues, and maybe even bones or other organs to get to the site of the tumor. The doses the tumor receives are also received by at least some of the adjacent normal tissue. Radiation causes damage to all cells it touches when given in high enough doses.

Some of the acute (faster-acting) side effects include breakdown of areas such as the skin and the mucous membranes (lining of the mouth, intestines, bladder), fatigue, nausea and vomiting, and swelling. Many patients actually appear to have been "sunburned" by their radiation therapy and require skin treatments to help with the local reactions. When significant radiation is given to a site such as the neck or face, the mouth can develop severe ulcers, pain, and decreased saliva production, and there can be difficulty in opening the jaw. This makes eating and drinking quite difficult, so many young patients need other interventions to help them get required nutrition. If someone's skull is radiated, they are likely to have hair loss in the area of the radiation. Unlike hair loss associated with chemotherapy, however, this hair loss is usually permanent but localized to the site that actually received the radiation. If the spinal cord or brain is treated, nausea and vomiting are more likely to occur. Side effects depend on the location of the radiation given.

There also are many side effects that are not noticeable during the radiation therapy and may appear weeks, months, and even years after the treatments are complete. If a salivary gland (a gland in the face responsible for producing saliva) gets irradiated, it probably will not function well in the future. People with radiation to this area will often have lifelong problems with dry mouth. Similar things apply to the eyes—if the eyes receive significant radiation, they are unlikely to produce tears in a normal fashion, and patients will need to use artificial tear drops indefinitely. Any tissue in the body (skin, muscle, lungs, etc.) that gets exposed to radiation treatments is at risk for something called fibrosis, where the tissue loses its elasticity or stretchiness and becomes harder to move.

In pediatric patients, radiation also will significantly affect the growth in the areas treated. A past example of a significant problem related to this is Wilms' tumor (tumor of the kidneys). Wilms' tumor usually affects only one kidney but often spreads within the abdomen and requires radiation treatments. At one time, patients received radiation to the side of the abdomen that the tumor came from. By irradiating only the one side, however, muscles and tissues on the other side of the body continued to grow, thus causing the spine to bend significantly to one side (severe scoliosis). Now, radiation oncologists make sure to include the spine and a certain portion of the other side of the abdomen in the radiation field to help keep the child's growth symmetric and prevent future problems with scoliosis. In another example, if a patient has a tumor in her leg that needs to be treated with radiation, that leg will not grow as well as the other, and the child will have an uneven leg length.

One of the most serious side effects of radiation is the development of another type of cancer later on in life. Children are more at risk for this problem than adults because their tissues are still involved in so much growth and they have so much more time to live than most adults who are treated similarly. These secondary cancers tend to occur many years after the initial treatment was given. Imagine a 65-year-old lady with breast cancer who received radiation and a 15-year-old teenager with Hodgkin's lymphoma who also received radiation treatments. If a secondary is likely to occur in 20 or 30 years after the radiation exposure, the 15-year-old is much more likely to have a problem down the road than the 65-year-old.

# OTHER LONG-TERM EFFECTS OF RADIATION THERAPY

Picture a child who is having a bone marrow or stem cell transplant to treat his leukemia. In many cases like this, the child is treated with total body irradiation (TBI), which helps clear his bone marrow of any leukemia cells. While this child is not treated with extremely high total doses of radiation, the manner in which this radiation is given is rather intense and concentrated over a short period of time. Since the whole body receives some dose of radiation, the child is at significant risk for many long-term effects.

For example, he could develop a secondary cancer of any part of his body, from the brain to the feet. Other effects are localized to particular areas, such as the head and neck. He is at risk for developing cataracts and other vision problems, so he should receive yearly ophthalmology exams. There is a risk for hearing loss, so his hearing should be screened at some point after treatment. His sinuses could develop inappropriately, and sinus infections could happen more frequently. Dry eyes and dry mouth might occur from damage to the fluid-producing glands in the head and neck. His teeth are likely to be damaged, so frequent visits to the dentist are important. The thyroid gland in the neck is especially sensitive to radiation, so he may develop thyroid disease or thyroid cancer later in life and should have yearly thyroid labs and examinations.

Patients who receive significant amounts of radiation to the brain are at risk for other complicated disorders. In general, if brain cells receive radiation, they are not going to function as well as they once did, so many children have some degree of loss of mental function. This can manifest as a drop in IQ (intelligence quotient) points, or as increased difficulty with certain types of schoolwork. Younger patients are more likely to experience significant problems than older patients who receive the same amount of radiation therapy.

Another key physical system that is controlled by the brain is hormone regulation (field of endocrinology). Many different hormone systems can be affected by radiation to the brain, including growth hormones, sex hormones, and steroid production. Some children require growth hormone replacement following brain irradiation. Others experience precocious puberty (puberty begins at too early an age), while still others experience pubertal delay or pubertal failure (puberty will not begin without medical intervention). When these problems occur, patients are usually referred to an endocrinologist who specializes in these medical issues.

In the chest and abdomen, several important organs are at risk from the treatment. The lungs may become less flexible from the radiation, so the lung function should be assessed periodically. The heart muscle may have a radiation effect as well, so frequent heart examinations are required. Women are at risk for poor breast development, and both men and women are at risk for breast cancer later in life. The liver and intestines may suffer some problems from the radiation as well. Both women and men are at risk for infertility as well because of radiation given to the gonads (ovaries or testes).

Of course, no one is expected to have all of these problems after radiation treatments, but the risks are there. One of the most important ways to counter these effects is to be vigilant about changes in the body and to take preventative measures such as routine blood work assessments and physical exams. There are an increasing number of special clinics dedicated to treating patients who are cancer survivors, helping them to lead more normal and healthier lives.

# Chapter 11

⤬

# STEM CELL AND BONE MARROW TRANSPLANTS

⤬

Some children and adolescents with cancer need something other than the basic surgery, chemotherapy, or radiation. These patients may be referred by the oncologist to a bone marrow transplant physician, who is usually another pediatric oncologist specializing in transplant therapy. The patient will first meet this specialist during a consult visit, where the transplant physician will collect details about the patient's medical and cancer treatment history, and will give the patient an overall sense of how the transplant process will affect him. During the initial or subsequent visits, the transplant specialist will require a lot of blood work and other types of tests to ensure that the patient is in the best health possible before pursuing this type of treatment.

A bone marrow transplant (BMT) or stem cell transplant (SCT) is a form of cancer therapy that is used fairly frequently in the treatment of pediatric cancers. When most people think of a "transplant," they imagine a surgical procedure where one organ is surgically taken from one person and then surgically put into another, much like what happens in kidney or liver transplants. However, a BMT/SCT is a relatively *non*-surgical procedure, and after experiencing it many people think the whole bone marrow infusion process is a bit anti-climactic.

A BMT/SCT is performed when a patient needs a very intense treatment to kill off the cancer cells in her body. One of the major side effects of this very intense therapy is depression of the patient's bone marrow, making the patient incapable of keeping her blood counts up without lifelong transfusion support. Bone marrow transplants, however, allow the patient's bone marrow, or stem cells, to make their own blood cells once again.

The donor, the person giving the stem cells to the patient, varies depending on the patient's type of cancer and his specific bone marrow type. In leukemia, it is better, in general, to give a patient someone else's bone marrow, because you want to give the patient cells that are free of leukemia. Even in the best of circumstances, you run the risk of returning leukemia cells to the patient if you give him back his own bone marrow cells. In solid tumors, since the cancer does not involve the bone marrow, it is better to use the patient's own bone marrow, which is "harvested" before the patient receives the intense treatment.

## AUTOLOGOUS TRANSPLANTS

An autologous transplant is one that involves the patient's own bone marrow (*auto* = self). These transplants are usually done in patients with solid tumors, such as neuroblastoma, Ewing's sarcoma, or medulloblastoma. In these transplants, the patient has a solid tumor that needs intense chemotherapy and/or radiation therapy to defeat the cancer. Knowing this, the physician will perform a "stem cell harvest" on the patient before she receives this intense chemotherapy, storing the stem cells until a time when they are needed. This harvest usually involves having a larger central line in the patient, from which the providers can take some of the patient's blood and selectively remove the stem cells, which are the precursor, or parent cells, to the rest of the cells in the blood. Occasionally, the physician is unable to get enough of the parent cells from the patient via the large IV, so the patient has to have the bone marrow procedure performed in the operating room, where the physician will do multiple bone marrow aspirates on the patient in order to get a good cell sample. These cells are later processed and saved to be re-infused into the patient after the intense treatment is given.

## ALLOGENEIC TRANSPLANTS

An allogeneic transplant is one that involves someone else's bone marrow (*allo* = other). These transplants are usually performed in patients who have cancers that involve their bone marrow, such as leukemia and some types of lymphoma. In these patients, once the provider decides that they need a transplant to give them a chance of a cure, the provider starts searching for an appropriate bone marrow donor. Donors range from family members to complete strangers. The process for determining who is an appropriate donor can be quite complicated. Once a donor is chosen, they can donate in a couple of ways. After the donor's bone marrow has been stimulated to grow and produce more cells by certain types of medications, the provider needs to collect stem cells or bone marrow from the donor. The donor will either have a large IV placed so that the physician can remove some of the donor's blood and have the precursor, or parent cells separated from the blood, or the donor can be taken to an operating room setting and have multiple bone marrow aspirates performed to obtain enough bone marrow product for processing and later infusion into the patient. (The bone marrow aspirate procedure is discussed in a separate chapter). Unlike regular bone marrow aspirates, though, the donor usually is given general anesthesia to ensure that he is completely asleep for the procedure. The procedure can be somewhat painful afterwards, because the provider has to perform the procedure many times at once. As with autologous transplants, the cells are later processed and saved for infusion into the patient.

The last classification of stem cell transplant is the syngeneic (*syn* = same) transplant, where the donor is actually the patient's identical twin. Syngeneic transplants, like autologous transplants, are typically more effective in solid tumor diseases than in leukemias, and the process of the transplant is similar to the allogeneic transplant.

## GRAFT VERSUS HOST DISEASE AND THE BEST DONOR FOR THE PATIENT

One of the major side effects or long-term complications of a transplant is called graft versus host disease, or GVHD. GVHD occurs because of an immune response that happens after the transplant has taken effect. The cells that were infused into the patient are the "graft," and the patient becomes the "host" for the cells. Sometimes, the infused cells (graft) start having an immune reaction against the patient (host), which can lead to significant side effects. Common sites of GVHD are the skin, liver, and gastrointestinal tract. Certain types of transplants are more likely to have problems with GVHD, and many transplant physicians are searching for better ways to prevent this complication.

Autologous transplants have no GVHD risk, because the graft and the host are part of the same immune system. Any allogeneic transplant can have a risk of GVHD, but the closer the match between the donor and the patient, the less risk of having this problem. When deciding on a bone marrow or stem cell donor for a cancer patient, the physicians look for the best match.

The matching process is based on a process called HLA (Human Leukocyte Antigen) typing, which is performed on a blood sample of the patient and the potential donor. Unlike routine blood typing for simple blood transfusions, the process of HLA-typing is much more complex and usually takes days to complete. These antigens are found on the surface of white blood cells, and the most common ones that are checked are HLA-A, -B, and -DR. Each person has two sets of these HLA groups, each inherited as a group from his mother and father. When people refer to a "six out of six match," the patient and the donor match on both groups of HLA-A, -B, and -DR. Some physicians look for patients to match on more areas than just the previous six antigens and will want patients and donors to be a "ten out of ten match."

A sibling who matches the patient is usually the best allogeneic donor. Any given sibling has a 25 percent chance of matching another full sibling. Each parent has two sets of HLA groups that he or she could pass on to any one child, so it's really a coin flip as to which group gets passed on to a given child. The sibling that is a full match has inherited both of the same groups of HLA antigens from each of the parents. A sibling that matches the patient is better than an unrelated donor, because the sibling is more likely to have other smaller antigens match the patient and have less problems with GVHD.

When a patient does not have a full sibling or does not have a sibling match, her physician will run a "marrow search," searching different marrow registries, looking for someone in the world with a similar HLA-typing to the patient. Some people have many potential matches found in the registry, while others may not have any match. It is typically more difficult for minorities or mixed-race individuals to find a good match, because that pairing of HLA sets is harder to find. Also, in the United States there are fewer minority volunteer donors in the national registry, making it harder for minority patients to find a match within America. Often, marrow registry programs will allow minority patients to register for free, hoping to boost the number of potential matches for these patients.

Once the transplant physician selects a potential donor from the registry, that person has to be contacted to see if he will actually be a donor. There are some people who forgot that they registered to be a donor, and they are not prepared to take on the responsibility of donating their bone marrow. Others may just get cold feet. Even if a potential transplant match agrees to be a donor, he must past a battery of tests, ensuring that he does not have any serious health problems or infectious diseases that could harm the patient receiving his marrow. It realistically can take several months to locate, prepare, test, and obtain a bone marrow specimen from a potential donor, which in some cases is too late.

An alternative for patients who have no suitable match in the marrow registries is a parent donor. Some centers believe that these "haploidentical" (half-match) donors are a good option for transplant in patients without other good options. Since each parent has given his or her child one set of HLA antigens, they are guaranteed to match at least half of the important sites nearly perfectly. Transplant physicians tend to process this marrow a little differently than they would someone who is a full match, and for some children this is the best option available.

## CORD BLOOD PRODUCTS

Umbilical cord products are another source of stem cells for a patient needing transplant. There are several places in the country and around the world that store umbilical cord samples after infant delivery for future medical purposes. Cord blood has some advantages over other donors; it is less likely to be infected with certain illnesses that could harm the patient, it tends to have higher numbers of the desired stem cells than regular adult blood, and it is usually more readily obtained than bone marrow from a grown person. Cord blood products also seem to have less risk of GVHD, so some providers will accept a cord blood product that is less of a match for the patient than a regular bone marrow specimen. However, some people worry about genetic illnesses that people could get from cord blood products. The infant that the cord blood came from could develop a serious illness in the early part of life, and since the cord blood products no longer have a link to the infants they came from, there is a theoretical risk that patients receiving these products could end up with other serious illnesses as a result of the transplant.

## PREPARATIVE OR CONDITIONING REGIMENS

Once the donor for the patient is secured and the product is being prepared, the patient starts receiving the intense therapy needed to conquer the cancer. This regimen is often called the preparative or conditioning regimen, which usually consists of some form of intense chemotherapy, with or without radiation therapy, depending on the age of the patient and the cancer being treated. The purpose of this regimen is to clear the body of any cancer cells and to weaken the body's immune reaction against the stem cells that will be infused. Most transplants done in children with cancer are myeloablative, meaning that they ablate the white blood cells in the patient's immune system.

Some of the more common chemotherapeutic agents used in these conditioning regimens are cyclophosphamide and busulfan. In older children and adolescents, these regimens often contain total body irradiation (TBI) as well. The TBI is split up over several days, often with twice daily treatments. The entire preparative regimen is usually started a few days in advance of the stem cell or bone marrow infusion. Patients will usually remain in the hospital from the time that the conditioning regimen begins until they have recovered their blood counts after the stem cell infusion, which typically takes a few weeks.

## THE TRANSPLANT ITSELF

On day "0," the patient receives her new stem cells, which typically take a couple of weeks to find their way to the bone marrow to start up a new blood cell immune system. The infusion of the stem cells is typically a short process, and one of the things that most people remember about the procedure is the smell. During the preparation process in the lab, the cells have to be carefully preserved, usually in dimethyl sulfoxide (DMSO). This DMSO has a very distinct smell when the product is infused into the patient and can cause even the toughest people some amount of nausea. The patient's vital signs (blood pressure, pulse, respiratory rate, temperature) are closely monitored during the infusion as well. After the infusion is complete, the patient usually does fairly well for the immediate future.

The effects of the preparative regimen are felt soon thereafter, with one of the biggest problems being mucositis. The patients have inflammation and ulceration of their mucous membranes, which usually has the worst effect on the oral cavity and intestines. While this side effect is not life-threatening, it is extremely painful, and patients will usually require high doses of narcotics to get them through these days. Children will also often refuse to eat because of the pain, so physicians will start patients on total parenteral nutrition (TPN), which is essentially nutrition by vein.

Physicians will also carefully monitor patients for infection, making sure to treat fevers and suspicious symptoms with strong antibiotics. Bacterial, viral, and fungal infections can each be life-threatening in patients. The best way to rid the body of the infection is through the immune system's white blood cells, but since these patients are waiting for working white blood cells, the antibiotics must work on their own to treat the patient.

Another serious and life-threatening complication that can occur after a transplant is veno-occlusive disease, or VOD. This is a severe liver injury noted by high levels of bilirubin, enlargement of the liver, and fluid retention. Blood flow within the liver is decreased, and the effects on the liver can be permanent.

While waiting for the new marrow to start working, patients usually need transfusion support; they require frequent red blood cell and platelet transfusions to keep their levels in a safe range. Labs will be checked at least daily to ensure that patients have normal blood counts and normal electrolyte levels while they are recovering. The most important sign of recovery is the return of the white blood cell counts, because this means that the donor infusion has finally found its way to the patient's bone marrow and is functioning as it should.

Occasionally, a patient experiences graft failure, in which the donated cells never find their way to the marrow. This patient must receive another stem cell infusion, either from the same donor or a different one, to allow him to recover. Without a good graft or infusion taking place in the bone marrow, the patient will be dependent on red blood cell and platelet transfusions indefinitely and will likely die from infection.

## GVHD AND GRAFT VERSUS TUMOR EFFECT

During the first three months after the infusion, patients are at risk for acute (early-onset) GVHD. This disease usually involves parts of the body like the liver, intestines, and skin. Physicians will often treat patients with medicines, such as prednisone (a steroid medication), that suppress the immune system further to prevent GVHD from happening. Some acute GVHD can be life-threatening, depending on the severity of the reaction and the location of the problem. Severe GVHD of the skin can actually cause the body to look like a burn patient; the skin will slough off and leave raw areas behind, thus causing pain and increasing the risk of infection in the patient.

Acute GVHD can become a more chronic problem, and chronic GVHD is the most common cause of long-term problems in post-transplant patients. Again, patients must be treated with medications to suppress the immune system, such as steroids or cyclosporine. There are many other newer medicines being tried for this problem, but no "magic pill" has been found. Many patients will have to take medications for chronic GVHD issues for months or even years after the transplant is over.

Many physicians believe in a concept known as "graft versus tumor effect," where the donor cells (the graft) actually provide an immune response against the cancer that has been plaguing the patient. It has been shown that leukemia patients who have some form of GVHD will often have a lower risk of the leukemia returning in their bone marrow. The same immune response that is involved in GVHD is also involved in fighting the cancer cells. Some physicians actually want patients with difficult-to-treat cancers to have some amount of GVHD, because it will likely help them in the long run. Obtaining the right balance between the GVHD and the graft versus tumor effect can be difficult.

# Chapter 12 &

# COMMON SIDE EFFECTS

&

Almost all children undergoing treatment for cancer will experience at least one effect of the cancer or the treatment itself. Some of these conditions, such as fever and neutropenia or mucositis, become very familiar to families taking care of a child with cancer. Many of these complications are anticipated, with a fairly standard treatment plan in place.

## FEVER AND NEUTROPENIA

Nearly every child receiving significant chemotherapy for her cancer will experience "fever and neutropenia" at some point during her treatment. Neutropenia is the condition that occurs when the patient's white blood cell counts are decreased to the point where the body's immune system can't function effectively to fight off infections. Most families become familiar with the child's blood counts during the course of therapy, paying particular attention to the white blood cell count and the "ANC" (absolute neutrophil count). When a child's ANC number is less than 500, she is considered to be significantly neutropenic, and at the greatest risk for infection. This risk is increased in children who have a central line for IV access.

If a child with a central line has an elevated temperature (greater than 100.5 to 101.5 F, depending on the oncologist's preference), that child usually needs to be seen as soon as possible, regardless of the ANC. Even in the face of a normal ANC and fever, the healthcare providers will obtain a blood culture (looking for bacteria in the blood stream) and blood counts to make sure that the child is safe from infection. Often, the provider also will give the patient a dose of IV antibiotics just in case there are bacteria in the blood. A child with an ANC below 500 and a fever usually ends up staying in the hospital for a few days, getting IV antibiotics until doctors can attest that there is no sign of significant bacterial infection. Children in this situation also have to show that their white blood cell counts are increasing, meaning that their immune system is starting to recover, before being allowed to leave the hospital.

Most children dealing with fever and neutropenia have one or two fevers and spend 48 to 72 hours in the hospital getting antibiotic treatments. These children are often infected with a virus that can't be isolated, and they recover without difficulty. Other children grow a specific type of bacterium in their blood from the blood culture. When this happens, the doctors will choose appropriate antibiotics to treat the bacteria for a typical 10 to 14 day course. Some of this therapy may be given at home through an arrangement with a home health care company, which provides nursing expertise in the home setting, allowing the parents to administer the antibiotics themselves.

Occasionally, the child will continue to have fevers for days with no known source of infection. When this happens, oncologists often consult infectious disease specialists to determine the proper antibiotics for the child. They may give the child two or three different antibiotics to treat an unknown infection source. Sometimes they suspect a fungal infection, which requires special treatment with anti-fungal medications. The doctors may start performing tests such as CT scans or bone marrow tests when children continue to have fevers with no source in order to see if there are other reasons for the fevers.

When a child has to deal with these prolonged courses of fever, parents and physicians alike get very frustrated. The fevers make the children feel miserable, and when the child feels bad, the parent gets more anxious. It can be difficult to treat fevers in children undergoing cancer therapies because the physicians are more limited in what types of medicine they can use to reduce the level of the fever. Usually, an anti-pyretic (anti-fever) medicine will reduce a person's temperature by one or two degrees. If a child has a fever of 104 F, then acetaminophen may lower the fever to 102 F. Children with cancer typically should not take ibuprofen or other non-steroidal anti-inflammatory medications, because they can prevent the patient's platelets (which are usually greatly decreased while a child is neutropenic) from working effectively, putting the child at risk for bleeding. A child not fighting cancer could take ibuprofen, bringing the temperature down to 100 F, while the child battling low blood counts has to remain at 102 F and is much more uncomfortable.

Certain features about a child's active treatment plan put him at risk for certain types of infections. For example, a child receiving high doses of steroids or cytarabine (ARA-C) is at greater risk of having specific aggressive bacterial infections than someone who is taking only oral chemotherapy medications. Some patients seem to have recurrent infections, with bacteria growing in their blood stream each time they have a fever. In these instances, there may be a problem with the patient's central line. Sometimes the central line can become colonized with bacteria, contaminating the line in a way that antibiotics will never be able to clear the infection. These patients may need to have their central line replaced with a new, clean, infection-free line. Most physicians will try to treat with antibiotics as long as possible before putting the child through another surgical procedure, but sometimes the line replacement just can't be avoided. Other children may have chronic problems, such as chronic sinus infections, which put them at risk for other types of infections. Sometimes physicians will want to get a piece of "tissue," meaning taking a biopsy of a part of the body that may contain the source of infection. If the biopsy is successful, physicians can then discover what is causing the infection and select the best therapy for the child.

## MUCOSITIS

Mucositis is the inflammation of a person's mucous membranes. These mucous membranes are the "wet" tissue that is present throughout our bodies. Most of the time, mucositis is limited to the mouth and oral cavity. However, it can affect the eyes, the esophagus, the intestines, the bladder, and even the urethra in certain patients. Chemotherapy and radiation therapies can put the patient at risk for mucositis. Sometimes patients have co-infections of the inflamed tissue and some other infection such as thrush or herpes virus. When other infections are present, physicians will prescribe specific therapies directed against that infection to help ease some of the symptoms.

Most patients, however, have no coinciding infections—just significant ulcers in the mouth or other mucous membranes. When present, mucositis can keep a child from eating or drinking, leading to malnutrition and other serious consequences. The pain associated with mucositis can be significant. Many patients require narcotic therapies to help them cope with this problem. Children at particular risk are those who have had bone marrow or stem cell transplants.

There are ongoing studies looking at particular medications which can be given to prevent mucositis from occurring, but results of these studies are not yet available. In general, physicians start off with encouraging good oral hygiene for the patients, with soft brushes for the teeth and gentle flossing when possible. Some recommend oral care rinses to help keep the mouth clean and free from debris. Once mucositis has started, there are various "coating" therapies that can help with the pain. Some of these agents are gel-like substances that coat the mouth, protecting the sores from pain when the child eats or drinks. Others contain lidocaine or some other combination of liquid products meant to help alleviate the pain, again with the goal that the patient will be more comfortable eating and drinking.

When the mucositis becomes more significant, patients can experience abdominal pain, chest pain, and bleeding in the urine. All of these processes may require more aggressive pain management, such as IV narcotic treatments. If a patient has extensive mucositis, the breakdown in that tissue barrier puts the patient at risk for specific infections, which come into play in the child with fever and neutropenia as well as the child with mucositis. Some patients are not able to maintain their own nutrition when they have mucositis, so physicians have to supplement their nutrition through their IV, using TPN (total parenteral nutrition). The use of TPN is usually temporary until the mucous membranes start to heal.

## BLOOD TRANSFUSIONS

Blood transfusions are fairly common in the lives of many pediatric cancer patients. Red blood cells can be given to patients with anemia, and platelets can be given to those with thrombocytopenia. Transfusions are usually done only in settings where the child is truly at risk with significantly low blood counts.

Many people have concerns about infections being transmitted to a patient through a blood transfusion. The infectious risks are real, but they are minimal with the current standards of blood safety. Due to the fairly recent issues surrounding hepatitis and human immunodeficiency virus (HIV), the American Red Cross has changed its standards regarding who can and cannot donate blood. The blood also goes through an extensive infection testing process to help decrease the risk of infectious complications.

However, some people still are uncomfortable giving their child blood from a stranger, so they may request to give the child their own blood or blood from another relative. In theory, this idea is a good one, but in practice it has its problems. First of all, it is difficult to predict when a child is going to need blood. It takes several days to get a unit of blood collected from a specific individual, such as a parent, for a designated child. Sometimes the child can't wait that long for the blood to become available. Second, the blood that comes from relatives is often not as safe as the blood that comes from the general population, because many relatives are embarrassed to admit certain lifestyle practices that may preclude them from donating blood to the general population. Third, when a child has a type of cancer that may require a bone marrow or stem cell transplant it is actually harmful to expose them to the blood of another family member prior to the procedure, because it can affect the outcome of the transplant itself.

Before a child is given any type of blood product, the patient's legal guardian must provide consent for the transfusion. The consent forms give specific numbers regarding the risks of developing certain types of infections. Once the guardian has given the consent, the hospital blood bank looks through its inventory for the most appropriate match for the child, based on the child's blood type and size. Some children are too small to receive an entire unit of blood, so these units may be split into separate parts, saving the second half of the same unit for the child at a later date, thus limiting the child's exposure to different blood donors.

Some children require "pre-medication" prior to getting their blood product. The nurse may give the child diphenhydramine to prevent allergic reactions, or acetaminophen to prevent febrile reactions. Red blood cells are typically infused over a period of two to four hours, while platelets are often given faster, over a period of 30 to 60 minutes. The nurses will keep a close eye on the child during the blood transfusion to ensure that no unexpected reactions occur. In the event that a reaction does occur, the transfusion is stopped and the patient is closely monitored. The most common reactions are low-grade fevers and itching or rash.

The physician may request blood work after the transfusion is complete to see that the child's blood got the proper effect from the transfusion. It is not uncommon for some children to need blood transfusions daily during certain periods of their cancer treatment.

## AFTER THERAPY: DEALING WITH PHYSICAL AND EMOTIONAL LONG-TERM EFFECTS OF TREATMENT

With the number of pediatric and adolescent cancer survivors increasing significantly over the past few decades, the field of medicine is starting to pay more attention to the special needs of these individuals. There are now clinics specializing in the care of cancer survivors. These centers help with many of the long-term physical and emotional needs these patients have.

For most, the battle with cancer is over, but these patients often face many other difficult problems related to their initial cancer diagnosis and treatment.

It can be extremely difficult to transition from intense cancer treatment to "normal life." For many patients and their parents, finishing therapy can be almost as traumatic as the initial diagnosis. When a young person is diagnosed with cancer, the lives of the patient and his loved ones are turned upside down. The weeks are now filled with doctor's visits and intense treatments. Some children visit the oncology clinic or hospital 100 times or more during their treatment course. Once the treatment journey is over, many feel as though their support has been taken away. People want to be happy and relieved that the treatments are complete and that the patient is cancer-free, but there is always a fear of the future and the "what if . . . "

*I didn't know what to do with myself. I spent the last three years of my life focusing on getting Alex through his leukemia treatments. Now there was no more chemotherapy to give, no weekly blood samples or physical exams. The doctors told us to be happy that he's finished and to come back in a month for a "routine" visit. He was able to attend school for an entire month without missing classes. I was able to take some time for myself, just doing things that I wanted to do. But none of it felt right. I missed the security of the clinic and the hospital. Any physical complaint that Alex had sent me into a panic. I didn't want to call the doctor's office with every little concern, and I desperately wanted Alex to make it a whole month without being seen, but I was terrified. What if that knee pain wasn't from him playing soccer at school? What if the leukemia was back? Why did he have that bruise on his arm? Were his platelet numbers OK?*

*After the first few months passed, things got a little easier. The routine at home had changed. I didn't expect to go to the clinic all the time, and I felt a little better about home life in general, but I still worried if the leukemia was going to come back. I never really allowed my mind to relax. Will Alex ever really have a normal life? Will there be later problems from his treatments? Will he have school problems? How will all this treatment affect his adult life? The questions haunted me every day. I desperately wanted to be happy but I just couldn't let go. [Excerpt from a conversation with a mother of a child with leukemia.]*

If these concerns arise, the families should always discuss their questions with the doctors. Pediatric oncologists will, for the most part, be very sympathetic towards patients and their families, because they know that the fear doesn't end when the treatment ends. After treatments are over there are new issues that arise, such as removing the central line, stopping antibiotics, and re-immunizing children.

For the most part, patients will still be fairly frequent visitors to the oncology clinic during the first year or two after treatments are complete. Some children need to get imaging studies done every three to six months. Others need labs checked every month or so. After being "off therapy" for a couple of years, however, some basic long-term issues need to be addressed in most patients, related to the specific therapies that each child received.

The patient may have these long-term issues attended to by the regular pediatric oncologist. Some patients may be referred to centers that specialize in "late effects" of cancer therapy. Others receive this care through their primary care physician. Unfortunately, some patients will never receive this care for a variety of reasons—from not knowing that it is needed to not being able to afford this type of visit.

During a complete examination for the potential late effects of cancer therapy, the providers perform a thorough analysis of the patient's treatment history. The specific types and doses of each chemotherapy medication will be recorded; any radiation therapy received will be noted; surgical procedures also will be analyzed. Any problems that the patient experienced during treatment will be added into a treatment summary for the individual patient. The late effects analysis will determine what tests need to be performed at specific time intervals to ensure that the patient has the best possible long-term outcome from her cancer treatment.

## PHYSICAL LATE EFFECTS OF TREATMENT

From head to toe, there are potential long-term physical effects from many cancer treatments. These effects can be from intense chemotherapy and bone marrow transplants, or from something simple such as a blood transfusion. In general, though, patients who receive the most intense therapies are the ones who are most at risk for significant late effects and complications. Some of the more serious late effects of radiation therapy and bone marrow transplantation are discussed in other chapters. However, surgery and chemotherapy treatments have their own potential long-term problems.

### Surgery Related Long-term Effects

Whenever a patient has any type of surgery, complications in the location of the surgery can occur that may persist for months or years after treatment. Scars can be problematic for many children or adolescents, and sometimes surgical revision of the scar is necessary. Nerve damage may occur to the skin around the surgical site, so some patients may have different sensations in specific areas of their skin. When an area of the body such as the abdomen is operated on, there is a risk of scar tissue forming within the surgical site, which can cause problems later on. For example, a patient who has had a tumor removed from his abdomen may develop scar tissue around the intestines. The scar tissue may obstruct the intestines to the point where no food or liquids will pass, and another surgery must be done to remove the scar tissue (known as breaking down adhesions).

Surgeries done to arms or legs can cause problems with use of the area involved. For instance, if a tumor is removed from the upper arm, there may be muscle that doesn't function correctly, making it difficult for the person to use the arm normally. Some people actually require amputation of an arm or leg for treatment, and those people are at risk for long-term pain problems and prosthetic concerns. This is apart from the expected psychosocial issues of having to lose a limb and the impact loss of a limb has on daily activities.

*Janie was diagnosed with osteosarcoma when she was seven years old. She had a tumor in the bone of her right thigh, and the surgeons thought that she would do best with a procedure called "limb-salvage" procedure, where she had the tumor and a good part of the bone removed, and a long piece of metal was put in its place. The surgery was difficult, and it took her several months to be able to walk "normally." One thing that really bothered her about her leg was that she had to get the prosthesis re-sized a few times, and this procedure was quite painful. She basically had to learn how to walk all over again each time the leg was changed. Since she had her surgery done years ago, there are other ways that people can be treated now. Another child in the clinic with the same type of cancer was given a "growing" prosthesis, so he doesn't have to have all the extra surgeries to keep his legs the same length. [Excerpt from a conversation with a mother of a child with osteosarcoma.]*

*When the doctors told us that Casey might lose his leg because of his tumor, we were terrified. How can a four-year-old live a normal life without a leg? Of course the first priority was beating the cancer, but removing his leg—this seemed so extreme! The surgeons removed his leg a few inches above his knee joint. The first few weeks were really hard on everyone. He had to deal with the pain from the surgery and the idea that he couldn't get around the way he used to. For us, looking at our son without his leg was such an obvious reminder of the cancer that was trying to kill him.*

*After the leg healed, he was given an artificial leg to work with. We were amazed at how quickly he adjusted to this new reality. It seemed like no time at all before he was back to getting around anywhere by himself, walking, playing, and even running! No one could have made us believe how well he would actually do without his leg. [Excerpt from a conversation with a father of a child with Ewing's sarcoma.]*

Some surgeries for cancer therapy require removal of specific organs, such as the testis or kidney. Long-term effects are obviously related to the organ that is now missing. An example of this is Wilms' tumor, where typically one kidney is removed during the initial diagnosis and treatment. This leaves the patient with one fully functioning kidney that now has to do the job of two kidneys. The remaining kidney usually grows a little in size to help with some of the work, but it sometimes is unable to handle the job. Patients are then at risk for developing problems with their remaining kidney, such as losing protein in the urine or being unable to filter electrolytes in the urine appropriately. These patients should have a urinalysis test done once a year to look for any potential problems.

Obviously, any procedure done on the brain or spinal cord can have tremendous effects on an individual patient. Any disruption of the normal nerve fibers can have fairly significant long-term consequences. Patients may have behavioral issues or school learning problems. In spinal cord operations in particular, there may be loss of motor function or sensation in patients following the surgery. While these problems may not be fully repairable, in many cases the schools and the families can work with the patient to ensure that they get adequate help with tests and activities of daily living.

### Chemotherapy Related Long-term Effects

One of the most common late effects of cancer therapy in children is a problem with their teeth. Any patient that receives chemotherapy is likely to have poor dental enamel and weak teeth roots. The risks seem to be greater in patients who are younger at the time of treatment. All patients should get routine dental examinations and aggressive treatment to prevent significant problems. Many patients are at risk for sight or hearing problems as well. Children who receive significant amounts of steroids during their treatment or who undergo bone marrow transplantation are at risk for developing cataracts and should have routine eye examinations. Patients who are treated with certain chemotherapy agents such as cisplatin or carboplatin should have routine hearing evaluations to pick up any hearing problems related to their treatment.

In the chest region, certain chemotherapy agents are associated with problems with long-term heart function. These medications include doxorubicin, daunorubicin, mitoxantrone, and idarubicin. These chemotherapy agents can affect the way the heart pumps blood throughout the body, keeping the muscles from working as efficiently as they once did. Patients are also at in increased risk of having a heart attack or irregular heart beats related to treatment with these medicines. Patients who have received any amount of this medication should be evaluated on a routine basis by echocardiograms and electrocardiograms. If any changes appear, evaluation by a heart specialist (cardiologist) is indicated. Female patients who were once treated with one of these medicines should take special care when considering pregnancy. The increased blood flow in the body that occurs after a woman becomes pregnant can add work to a sometimes already stressed heart, making the pregnancy high-risk for the female and her unborn child. Obstetricians should be made aware of the prior chemotherapy exposure and should monitor the mother's heart function routinely throughout the course of pregnancy.

Another area that can be affected by chemotherapy medicines is the lung. The chemotherapy agents bleomycin and busulfan potentially can cause changes to the lungs called pulmonary fibrosis, in which the lungs are less elastic than they once were, making certain breathing activities more difficult. Patients treated with these medicines should be referred for pulmonary function testing (PFTs). During this test, the patient is asked to breathe through a tube into a machine that records the speed of air movement and amount of air in the lungs to see if the lungs are functioning properly. If abnormalities are noted, further testing may be required.

The abdomen and pelvis are home to many organ systems that can feel an effect from chemotherapy. The liver is a target of some of the chemotherapy agents used, but the effects on the liver are typically short-lived. Very rarely, a patient will have a long-term effect on the liver related to blood flow in the liver. This disorder is known as portal hypertension, and it has mostly been associated with the use of 6-TG, or thioguanine. With portal hypertension, the blood pressure in the portal vein (a vessel in the liver) is higher than the blood pressure in the hepatic veins (other liver blood vessels). The effects of portal hypertension are related to changes in blood flow, which is, in turn, related to the increased pressure in the portal vein. Since the portal vein needs extra force to make the blood go through it, the blood tends to be funneled into other blood vessels with less pressure. This causes the spleen to become large (splenomegaly) and leads to larger blood vessels in the esophagus. If this process continues for a significant amount of time, the patient may need aggressive treatment of this disorder.

The kidneys also can feel the effects of several different chemotherapy medicines over a long period of time. Medications such as cisplatin, carboplatin, and ifosfamide can affect how the kidneys filter items through the urine. In some patients, the kidneys will waste important electrolytes, such as magnesium and potassium in the urine. These patients have to take supplements of these electrolytes as treatment. Other patients develop high blood pressure or protein in their urine related to these treatments. Simple blood pressure screens and urine and electrolyte tests can detect these problems, steering patients towards appropriate treatment.

Patients who received cyclophosphamide or ifosfamide are at risk for having problems with their bladder, ranging from difficulty with urinating to extra fluid within the kidneys (hydronephrosis) to blood in the urine. Those who received higher doses of these medications are at greater risk for these complications. Any change in the urinating patterns or color in the urine should be investigated by the provider caring for the patient. A small group of patients who are treated with cyclophosphamide may also be at risk for developing cancer of the bladder later in life. Children and adolescents treated with this medication should get urine screens once a year for the rest of their lives, looking for changes in the urine that could be signs of this type of cancer.

One of the most difficult late effects of cancer treatment in children and young adults is infertility. It is extremely hard to tell the parents of a child that she may never be able to have children of her own. Of course, at the time that the child is receiving therapy, the most important goal is to cure the child of cancer. It is very hard to conceptualize fertility risks in a four-year-old, but people need to be aware of this potential risk of certain chemotherapy agents. Many different drugs are associated with this risk: busulfan, cyclophosphamide, ifosfamide, carboplatin, and cisplatin are just a few. The risk of problems seems to increase with the total dose of the medications, and males seem to have more problems than females. In males, the late effects include delayed puberty, low male sex hormones, low numbers of sperm, and complete infertility. In females, the risks include not only delayed puberty and infertility, but early menopause as well. Menopause in these women may occur in the 20s instead of the usual 40s or 50s age range. Fortunately, there are many advances happening in the field of fertility enhancement, and a lot of patients are able to take advantage of other options to allow them to have children. Families and physicians need to work to give post-pubertal males the chance to donate their own sperm and have it stored for later use prior to receiving any toxic chemotherapy treatments.

There are some other "body systems" that can feel the effects of chemotherapy as well. The bones are at particular risk, especially after treatment with steroids or certain forms of methotrexate. Patients may develop early osteoporosis or weakening of their bones unexpectedly, which puts them at risk for developing fractures and other bone complications later in life. Children who are treated with steroids are also at risk for a disorder called osteonecrosis, where the bone is affected by poor blood flow to the area, and essentially a small piece of bone dies, causing significant pain in the individual. Usually, this bone change happens during the early part of treatment, but in some people the symptoms may either progress or resolve with time.

Patients who received medications such as etoposide, busulfan, cyclophosphamide, ifosfamide, cisplatin, carboplatin, doxorubicin, daunorubicin, idarubicin, or mitoxantrone should have yearly blood tests performed for the first few years after therapy is complete. These children and adolescents are at special risk for developing another cancer, acute myelocytic leukemia (AML) within the first five to ten years after treatment. Those that received cisplatin and carboplatin are also at risk for developing high cholesterol levels, so they should have their cholesterol checked routinely.

Another area of concern for many cancer patients is their cognitive function. All patients, but especially young children who are exposed to certain chemotherapy agents such as cytarabine and methotrexate at high doses are likely to have some problems with school. The problems may be subtle, such as difficulty with organization or memory. However, many children have certain learning problems with math and reading comprehension that require extensive modification of assignments and testing situations. In most cases, the parents and the teachers can work together to find the best learning environment for the student. Some patients need limitations on the amount of homework given; others need tests without time restrictions. All things considered, though, there are many cancer survivors in the world who received these high dose treatments who are accomplished, intelligent, active members of society, with many outstanding achievements.

## SOCIAL AND EMOTIONAL LATE EFFECTS OF TREATMENT

Some of the most difficult long-term problems in patients with cancer are the emotional effects of therapy. Having cancer changes a person and his loved ones dramatically. In some, the process actually makes them stronger. For others, however, cancer is the beginning of an extremely difficult life, filled with anger and disappointment. Patients who have cancer are at risk for depression, anxiety disorders, and even post-traumatic stress disorder. They may have unexplainable pain from their prior therapies that affects their daily activities and lifestyle. Some become withdrawn and have difficulties functioning in society, while others rebel against society, getting involved in illegal activities or unsafe behaviors.

Certain individuals seem to be at greater risk for developing emotional problems after cancer treatment. Those who were adolescents or young adults at the time of diagnosis often have a harder time adjusting, not only to the cancer treatments themselves, but to the idea that they will always be different from those around them. Patients who have cancer treatments that affect their brain's function, such as chemotherapy given directly into the spinal fluid or radiation to the head, seem to have more difficulties handling the emotional stress. Those who require more intense treatments, such as bone marrow or stem cell transplant, or multiple rounds of chemotherapy treatments, may require a stronger social support system to get them through the issues and problems that they will likely face later in life.

One of the more difficult tasks for many cancer survivors is the return to school. While some children continue to attend school during their treatments, others rely on home-schooling for their education because of the need to spend so much time in the hospital setting. Once treatment is over, most patients will get back into the regular routine, which includes daily attendance at school. Children and adolescents often re-enter school with a sense of uncertainty, wondering how classmates, friends, and teachers will react. Many children receive support from their classmates during their time of treatment in the form of letters, cards, and even presents. This may help them feel more comfortable about returning to the classroom group because they know that they were not forgotten.

The response from many parents is to be overprotective. It can be very difficult to let a child go off to school at any point during therapy, and returning at the end of treatments is no easier. One way to "ease" children back into the classroom setting may be to arrange one-on-one play dates or outings with close friends who go to the same school. This will give the child a contact point when they return to full classes, and it may give them an idea of what types of questions other children will ask.

Most children and adolescents just want to fit in with their classmates. Having people know that they were sick from cancer makes them different, and being different is not always a good thing in a child's eyes. It is often helpful to meet with the school teachers and administrators prior to the first day back to help minimize the stress on the child. The cancer survivor should be prepared for whispers and looks on their return, especially if other students in the school know any details about why they've been gone. Being up front with others about the cancer diagnosis and treatments is often the best way to get past the initial strange feelings. However, once the initial adjustment has passed, it may become difficult to discuss healthcare issues with other students because it makes them feel uncomfortable. Unfortunately, this may only add stress to the patient, because they aren't free to talk about this important area of their life. Providing other outlets for the child to discuss the past diagnosis and therapies and the future concerns can be very helpful.

## PAYING FOR LATE EFFECTS OF TREATMENT

For many childhood cancer survivors, one of the more difficult hurdles becomes medical insurance coverage as an adult. Cancer is a very expensive illness. Without insurance, and even with insurance in some cases, treatment for cancer can lead to bankruptcy. As a child or teenager, most are covered under their parents' medical insurance policies, but most of these policies stop covering the patients once they get out of school or become adults. Getting replacement insurance under the name of the cancer patient can be very difficult, as almost all insurance companies have "pre-existing condition" clauses, and will not cover any treatments or care related to the prior diagnosis of cancer. In some cases, however, the pre-existing condition clause lasts for a set period of time, so if a patient is ten years from her treatment, she may be completely insurable.

Families and patients need to research insurance companies and their coverage policies years before the patient becomes an adult if at all possible. Sometimes it may be worthwhile to enroll on an insurance plan early so that the patient will be covered for any major illnesses immediately after the parents' insurance expires. If private medical insurance is unavailable, there may be some federally funded programs that can help cover any lapses in coverage. Again, investigating these options early is very important.

For many, the insurance issue becomes part of a vicious cycle. Some patients are too sick to work, and therefore too sick to tag onto an employer's insurance plan or pay for expensive insurance out of pocket. The medical care becomes more expensive, thus adding to the stress of the situation, and this further exacerbates the health problems of the patient. Knowing about potential resources such as low cost or free prescription programs and discounted or free health care clinics can be very helpful to these individuals. Often, a clinic or hospital social worker can lead someone in the right direction for getting affordable and adequate health care coverage.

# Chapter 13

## COMPLEMENTARY AND ALTERNATIVE MEDICINE IN CANCER

When faced with the diagnosis of cancer, many start wondering about the treatments that are being offered to them by the standard healthcare profession. The thought of using toxic treatments such as chemotherapy and radiation are terrifying for most families, and it is natural to want to find the perfect answer for cancer that won't expose a child to "unnatural" therapies. With easy access to the Internet, many people go searching on their own for the magic cure. Many "treatments" that are available include vitamin-based therapies, natural medicines, and non-medicine-based therapies.

Complementary and alternative medicine (CAM) is the term used to describe all of these different types of healthcare practices and products that are not part of more conventional medicine. Conventional medicine is defined as the currently accepted treatment for a specific disease based on the results of past research, and this is the medicine that is given in most hospitals in the United States. It includes the standard care provided by medical doctors (MD), doctors of osteopathy (DO), registered nurses, and physical therapists.

Complementary medicine is used in conjunction with conventional medicine. Alternative medicine is used instead of conventional medicine. There are many different types of CAM therapies available all over the world, and while some have merit, others may be designed merely to make money for individuals who are preying on the vulnerability of those in difficult situations.

The National Center for Complementary and Alternative Medicine (NCCAM) is a group run by the National Institutes of Health (NIH), and they have defined some major groups within the realm of CAM therapies:

### Whole Medical Systems

These are entire systems of medicine that were built outside of the medical approach used in the United States. These medical systems have their own specific practices and include naturopathic medicine, homeopathic medicine, and traditional Chinese medicine.

### Mind-Body Medicine

The main idea behind mind-body medicine is that the mind can affect the body, so by working to improve and enhance the mind, you can get better control over the body and the illnesses that afflict on the body. Some examples of this type of CAM are support groups, prayer, cognitive-behavioral therapy, and music therapy.

### Biologically Based Practices

These are mainly treatments using substances that are natural, such as vitamins, herbs, special foods, and other dietary supplements.

### Manipulative and Body-Based Practices

These CAM are related to actual movement or manipulation of different parts of the body, such as massage or chiropractic medicine.

### Energy Medicine

The group of energy medicine includes bioelectromagnetic-based therapies, such as magnetic fields, and biofield therapies, such as qi gong and Reiki. With any area of energy medicine, the basic idea is to affect the energy fields that are thought to surround the human body.

With nearly one-half of all pediatric cancer patients participating in some form of CAM therapy, this has become an important area in the treatment of children with cancer. These therapies can be used to counteract side effects and symptoms of more conventional therapies, and sometimes they are used to support patient healing. Another term for this type of treatment is Integrative Medicine (IM), which encourages the use of the patient's body, mind, and spirit together to enhance the cancer treatment. IM combines the use of conventional cancer therapies and some components of CAM therapy.

The Consortium of Academic Health Centers for Integrative Medicine (CAHCIM) was created in 2002, and it serves to use a science-based model of healthcare, using both conventional and scientifically-sound CAM therapies. These therapies are usually more readily available in large academic centers that treat adult cancer patients, but their use is becoming more common in pediatric patients as well. Many medical schools are also teaching some CAM therapies as part of the medical student curriculum.

Families interested in pursuing these complementary or alternative therapies need to understand that most of the time they are not covered by the medical insurance system. This is starting to change somewhat, but each person should check with individual insurance companies to see which practices, if any, are covered.

## CAM IN RESEARCH

The NCCAM is a federal agency that is working in scientific research on CAM. Its main goal is to look at all different types of non-conventional therapy and examine them as other conventional therapies are analyzed. Good, quality research in these areas is needed to see if there are alternatives to standard chemotherapy and radiation therapy that are useful in the field of cancer therapy. When it comes to pediatric cancer therapy, however, it is extremely difficult to get acceptable treatments for children. In most instances, as in conventional medicine, the therapy must show some benefit in adults before it can be tried for children.

Many people will research some type of CAM during their child's cancer treatment plan, and sometimes they will refuse conventional care and embrace this other form of treatment. Motivations for pursuing different types of treatments vary from person to person. However, most people need to find some area of control when they are caring for a child with cancer, and for some, researching other therapies, whether conventional or alternative, gives them a sense that they are participating in defeating their child's cancer.

When considering some form of alternative or complementary treatment for cancer, it is in the child's best interest to make sure that the oncologist also knows about these other treatments. Most pediatric oncologists are somewhat aware of some of the non-conventional medical options that are used by or sold to people with cancer, and sometimes the oncologists can help guide the family to safer options.

There are active clinical trials conducted through conventional health centers using CAM therapy. Some of these trials are looking at ways of using CAM treatments to boost the immune system or improve the effects of treatment. Others are looking at potential ways to reduce the risk of developing cancer. Patient families need to know that many pediatric oncologists are open to using an IM treatment for children along with conventional therapy. These physicians understand the need to keep the patient as healthy as possible from every aspect of his care.

Problems occur, however, when families refuse to continue with conventional therapies that are known to work to cure the cancer. There are many instances where families have refused chemotherapy or radiation therapy in hopes of finding a less toxic treatment elsewhere. Sometimes, patients are cured of their disease. Whether the cure comes from the alternative treatments is not fully known, and there is not one specific treatment that will cure all people. (These patients may already have received some benefit from conventional treatments before pursuing the alternative therapies, and the overall picture of what led to the cure becomes unclear.) More often, though, patients cannot be cured through these other therapies, and when they return for more conventional treatment, the cancer has become so advanced that cure is no longer an option.

## WHEN CAM THERAPIES ARE HARMFUL

Some CAM therapies can actually work against some of the treatments that the oncologist may be using to treat the cancer. An example is treatment with the chemotherapy agent, methotrexate. Methotrexate essentially works by depleting folic acid from the body. The cancer cells feel the effect of the lack of folic acid before the normal cells do, so they are killed first by the folic acid depletion. When needed, the doctor will use a medicine called leucovorin, which is a form of folic acid rescue, to save the normal cells in the body from feeling the effects of the lack of folic acid. Vitamins are one of the most common complementary treatments used by parents. Many parents think that vitamin supplements should be given to their child and that they can only help the body's defense against cancer. However, when the vitamin supplements contain folic acid, it makes the methotrexate therapy ineffective, eliminating one of the more useful forms of chemotherapy.

Acupuncture is a form of CAM therapy that is becoming more widely used in the United States. It has been used in Eastern cultures for centuries and has some real medical merit. Some more recent pediatric cancer trials have looked at incorporating acupuncture into the treatment regimens to help with chemotherapy-induced nausea and vomiting. This treatment has shown benefit for adults undergoing cancer therapy. In the setting of a conventional medicine treatment trial, though, the practitioner must meet certain training standards to give this care to a young child. When families look to find an acupuncturist from other sources, they must be careful in choosing the practitioner. The acupuncturist must be well trained (licensed in his field), and use disposable sterile needles. If the treatment is given improperly, the patient can develop infections, bleeding, or damage to internal organs.

There are other CAM therapies that may be harmful during cancer treatment. These include high doses of certain vitamins. Some vitamins, when taken in excess doses, can be toxic to anyone's system. These include the "fat soluble" vitamins, which are Vitamins A, D, E, and K. Fat soluble vitamins are stored in the liver and fat and are harder to eliminate from the body. Increased use of dietary antioxidants can also be harmful during treatments because they may interfere with chemotherapy and radiation therapy. Certain herbs, such as St. John's wort, may interfere with chemotherapy levels as well and can actually cause the body to feel the toxic effects of chemotherapy more because of its interaction.

A parent needs to make sure that any CAM therapy they are considering for their child is safe. While the Internet is a great source for information, it also can be full of misleading information. There is a database available on PubMed, called CAM. This was developed by the National Library of Medicine and the NCCAM. This database provides information about scientific studies that have been done using different types of CAM.

Some people would prefer to use a Web site that discusses the specific CAM treatment as their main source of information. When using a Web site, the user must be wary of the information given. Parents need to keep in mind the purpose of the site (education or sales), the sponsor of the site (reputable source, drug manufacturer, etc.), and how current the information is.

Some key words that are often used on Web sites describing CAM therapies need to be viewed cautiously. One such word is "natural." Many people see natural, and think that the product must be safer for them to use. This is not always the case. This is extremely important when looking at specific therapies, such as dietary supplements. Dietary supplements have no government regulation for the source of the ingredients, how much of the ingredients are included, or the quality of the manufacturing process. The U.S. Food and Drug Administration (FDA) has no jurisdiction over dietary supplements, and just because a supplement is described as natural, does not mean that it is safe.

When a CAM product sounds too good to be true, it probably is. One should be wary of products that claim to cure many different diseases. Most products that are worthwhile are suitable to treat or take care of one or two particular medical issues. It is very difficult to believe that a single treatment can cure diabetes, cancer, pain, and depression all at the same time. If a product were truly that effective, it is unlikely that it would be found only on a small Web site.

## INFORMATION ABOUT SELECTED TYPES OF CAM THERAPIES

There are literally hundreds of potential CAM therapies available for use. A few of the more common treatments are discussed here.

### Acupuncture

Acupuncture has been used as a part of traditional Chinese medicine for thousands of years. Its use in the United States has been limited to the past 200 years, and the U.S. Food and Drug Administration approved the use of the acupuncture needle as a medical device in 1996. The process of acupuncture involves the application of needles, pressure, heat (moxibustion), or other treatments to areas on the skin known as acupuncture points. Most people in the United States are familiar only with the needle form of the treatment. Its main role in cancer therapy has been to relieve some of the nausea and vomiting caused by chemotherapy. There have been many studies, both in animals and humans, which suggest that acupuncture may truly be beneficial in the treatment of nausea. Acupuncture has also had some role in treating cancer-related pain.

To become an acupuncturist, the practitioner has to go through a strict training and licensure program. The number of licensed acupuncture providers in the United States has been increasing in recent years. These trained professionals are very stringent in how they provide the service. One key feature to a safe procedure is the use of disposable/single-use needles for each patient. Without this technique, patients can be exposed to many different infectious blood-transmitted illnesses.

### Aromatherapy

In aromatherapy, people use the essential oils from plants to produce physiologic effects. These oils can be inhaled or placed directly on the skin to get their effect. Some of the more common oils include lavender, chamomile, and cedarwood. This therapy has few, if any, harmful side effects, and many believe that some of the oils can have either calming or energizing effects on the person using them.

The molecules are said to have an effect on the emotional center of the brain, the limbic system. Each molecule can have a different effect on the limbic system. Scientists have looked at the brain through functional imaging studies (tells how the brain is working during a therapeutic treatment), and these studies support the idea that these aroma molecules may provide a real benefit.

## Qigong

Qigong was originally used as part of traditional Chinese medicine. This technique is often taught with certain Chinese martial arts. In general, qigong is done to help maintain good health through various physical postures and motions of the body combined with different breathing patterns. There are many different forms of qigong. This technique is related to the idea that the body has something like an energy field that is kept in check by the breath of the body. The word qi means breath or gas in Chinese. Gong means work applied to a discipline. This "breath work" helps a person manage breathing to allow her to remain in good health and enhance the body's stamina.

This technique has been used as a standard medical treatment in China since 1989 and is taught in major Chinese universities. It has been included in Chinese health plans since 1996. However, the benefits to qigong in these settings typically surround its use to maintain a person's health through appropriate exercise and improved joint flexibility. Others have made claims that qigong can provide a greater benefit through actually healing an individual of her disease, but these claims have not been scientifically proven.

## Massage Therapy

Many people use massage therapy as an adjunct to medical treatments. It has been in use for thousands of years in many different cultures. It became more widely used in the United States in the 1800s, and has seen a resurgence in popularity over the last 40 or 50 years. Sometimes it is used as a specific treatment, but it is more commonly used to promote general wellness. Massage therapy has few associated risks when performed by licensed, trained massage professionals. The individual therapist's training affects the type of massage delivered, as all massages are not alike.

Trigger point massage, or pressure point massage, focuses on specific knots in the muscles which can be trigger points for discomfort. Deep tissue massage focuses on the muscles which are deep under the skin and involves muscles stroking and deep finger pressure. Shiatsu massage uses a rhythmic pressure by the fingers on specific areas of the body to help with the individual's energy. Swedish massage works to help with joint flexibility by using kneading, stroking, and friction on the muscles.

There are several ways in which massage may benefit a cancer patient. For those dealing with pain, it is thought that massage therapy may help block some of the pain signals that get sent to the brain. It can be helpful in leading a person to be well-rested, which can be better for their overall health. It may also be beneficial in sleep patterns for patients who have difficulty sleeping.

There are only a few conditions which should lead a person to avoid massage therapy. These include blood clots, damaged blood vessels, or bleeding disorders, as well as weakened bones or acute illness or infection. Patients with cancer may be at particular risk for some of these conditions, so it is wise to discuss the risks and benefits of massage with the healthcare provider prior to initiating any sort of massage therapy.

# Chapter 14
## CHOOSING AMONG POTENTIAL TREATMENTS

Being faced with cancer is a life-altering event for anyone. Parents are put under a lot of pressure to make a choice about their child's treatment. The parents are often the ultimate influence on what therapy will be given to their child. How can a parent or guardian know that the treatment they choose will be the best? If their child has problems with treatment, how does a parent reconcile the guilt that they may feel about what may have been the wrong choice?

The course of cancer therapy is filled with many choices. Oftentimes, the first choices are the most difficult and the most important. How and when should I tell my child the truth about her illness? What type of treatment will be used to cure the cancer? Should I allow a central line to be placed in my child? If so, what type of line? Sometimes the child's caregivers disagree about the way the child should be treated. The mother and father may feel comfortable with the care that the doctor is recommending, but family members may be distrustful of the medical system and insist that the parents look elsewhere for therapy. One of the most difficult situations is when the parents disagree with each other. One parent may want to be aggressive with the therapy and push for chemotherapy and radiation treatments early on, while the other parent wants to wait and see how the child does before jumping into a potentially devastating therapy.

*Lindsey never liked doctors. At two years of age, every time we took her in to see the doctor she screamed and fought the entire time. We got to where we just quit taking her in to the clinic. Her father and I made sure that she ate healthy and stayed away from food products and chemicals that could harm her. She was almost never exposed to sick children, and she never needed any antibiotics. It was extremely difficult for us when she developed a fever and this horrible cough and couldn't breathe right. We broke down and took her to the doctor. After they examined her, they recommended an X-ray of her chest to see if she had pneumonia. Instead of pneumonia, though, it showed a large mass that was pushing on her windpipe.*

*The next few hours were a whirlwind. She was poked and prodded and put through many horrible tests that made her so upset. They finally told us that she had some type of leukemia, and the mass in her chest was part of her leukemia. This mass was making it very difficult for her to breathe, and she needed immediate treatment if she was going to live. The doctors said that she had to get radiation to her chest to keep this mass from completely closing her windpipe, and this radiation had to be given as soon as possible.*

*I didn't want her to get the radiation. How could radiation help treat her? She couldn't have leukemia—we were so careful with her, watching what she ate and did, never letting her be exposed to something dangerous to her body or her spirit. Now this doctor is telling us that she needs to be radiated? Radiation causes cancer. Radiation could never be good for Lindsey. My husband disagreed with me. He wanted Lindsey to get the treatment right away. He didn't seem to care that we were going to expose our child to all this radiation. I was amazed that he could think that radiation was a good thing. I absolutely refused, and he insisted that she be given the treatment. It was the toughest moment in our relationship at one of the most critical times in our daughter's life. [Excerpt from a conversation with a mother of a child with leukemia.]*

Many parents believe they have *no* choice in regard to their child's cancer treatment. Depending on the emotional state of the parent, this can be helpful or harmful. Some parents feel a trust in their child's doctor, and whatever that doctor recommends is what they will do. This is especially true at the beginning of treatment, when things have to happen fairly quickly and it is hard to question proposed therapy. Other parents prefer to question everything. Sometimes these parents have a strong medical background and knowledge base. Or, they may have had bad experiences in the medical system and become distrustful of what they believe are hasty recommendations. Each type of family offers its own challenges for the oncologist treating the child, whose main goal is to rid the child of his cancer.

Pediatric oncologists in general want families to understand as much as possible about their child's care. Many of these parents feel like they should have earned a medical degree by the time the cancer treatment is over, because they've learned so much about this area of medicine. When families tell the doctor "whatever you think is best," the doctor still wants the family to be comfortable and understand why a particular therapy is being chosen. Families who question everything are most likely to get detailed explanations about treatment plans, with the intent of convincing them that the proposed treatment is the best one for their child.

## STANDARD TREATMENT OPTIONS

For most patients, standard cancer treatments include some combination of surgery, chemotherapy, and/or radiation therapy. Most pediatric oncologists will present families with a plan, or "roadmap," of their treatment that outlines the expected treatment course. This roadmap allows families to have a timeline of upcoming treatments, including specific chemotherapy infusions, lab testing, radiology studies, and radiation treatments (when applicable). Some of these roadmaps include treatment plans that extend for a couple of years, whereas others only cover a span of weeks to months.

Each page of the roadmap may represent a different phase of therapy. The plan includes each type of chemotherapy agent and the date it is due to be given. This plan is like a calendar, allowing the doctors to keep track of when specific studies need to happen and when the child will have to be hospitalized for treatment. Sometimes, patients get "off-schedule," usually related to unexpected side effects of therapy. Other times, the patient is deliberately moved from the planned treatment dates for non-medical reasons. One reason might be a special event that the child wants to attend, like a birthday celebration or school dance. Other reasons may include holiday celebrations, important family trips, or long-awaited vacations. In most cases, the doctors can be somewhat flexible with the schedule for these important circumstances.

The details of the chemotherapy administration vary, depending on the type of cancer, the type of chemotherapy, and the patient's overall health status. Surgery will also vary from patient to patient. Leukemia patients will likely have little interaction with the surgeon except for placement of a central line, while osteosarcoma patients rely heavily on the surgeon's skill and expertise. Naturally, the type of surgery depends on the type and location of the tumor. Only a small portion of pediatric cancer patients will actually require radiation therapy, and the details of this therapy again depend on the type and location of the cancer. Further information regarding all three types of standard cancer therapy is provided in other sections.

## ALTERNATIVE TREATMENT OPTIONS

On occasion, families will have strong beliefs that the standard medical care offered in the United States does more harm than good. The idea of putting poisons in a child to treat cancer is horrific to them, and they want to look elsewhere for therapy. As discussed in the "alternative" therapies section, there are many places throughout the world that offer "miracle" cures for cancer. While many are skeptical of these claims, it is natural for a parent to want to find the perfect cure for this horrible illness—something that will get rid of the disease but will not cause any direct harm to the patient while getting to the cure. Unfortunately, there is no perfect cure yet, either with standard therapies or alternative ones.

Most families choose to pursue the standard treatment options offered to their child. Some of these families also pursue complementary treatments that are offered elsewhere to aid in the fight against cancer. These complementary treatments usually seem to focus on nutrition and its role in treating cancer. Parents may start their children on nutritional supplements purchased on the Internet or in stores, or they may follow recipes given to them for cancer treatments. In general, these supplements are not harmful to the child. However, it is safest to let the child's oncologist know exactly what you are giving her. Provide them with labels or bottles when applicable. This way the doctor can determine if there are any dangerous interactions between the nutritional therapies and the standard medical therapies being used.

If a family wishes to pursue a complementary treatment for their child's cancer, and the patient's doctor has a closed mind about this practice, the physician-family relationship can become strained. Many parents view this as a lack of respect for their wishes, and it can cause them to lose respect for the medical provider. It is in the child's best interest for family and physician to communicate about all treatments that are being given. This will help keep them safer during their intense therapy.

There have been instances, often well-publicized, when parents altogether refuse any standard medical care for their child with cancer. When a child has a more easily treatable form of cancer, such as Hodgkin's lymphoma or acute lymphoblastic leukemia (ALL), the physicians may feel that the refusal of standard care is equivalent to child maltreatment. If a child has a proven 85 percent chance of cure from his cancer by pursuing a standard treatment, and certain death by doing nothing, the physician will do everything possible to give the child the standard treatment. There have been cases where physicians and hospitals have taken parents to court over this matter, even having the children removed from parental custody to give them the best chance of survival. In instances where the chance of survival is so high with standard treatment, the court usually sides in favor of the medical system. Sometimes the overall survival for a specific cancer case is less clear, and the courts may decide to rule in favor of the patient's parents. While this whole scenario is unfortunate, there are times when the families and physicians cannot come to an agreement about the best care for the patient, and these extreme measures become necessary.

## OTHER CANCER TREATMENT CHOICES

Some parents and patients face an extremely difficult decision during therapy for tumors of the arms or legs. In bone tumors such as Ewing's sarcoma and osteosarcoma, they may be offered a choice of limb-sparing surgery or amputation. In the limb-sparing surgery, the surgeon replaces the bone with something else. It can be another bone of the patient's, a bone from someone else, or a mechanical prosthesis. With amputation, the patient loses that portion of her body permanently, but in many instances an external prosthesis can be developed to replace the limb that was lost during the surgery. Both procedures have their own risks and benefits, and their own long-term problems.

When faced with a treatment option like this, families should be given extensive information about each option. They should take the time to talk about the options with friends, family members, and the child affected by the surgery. Another helpful option is to find someone else who has been through a similar procedure. Parents can ask the doctors to refer them to another family or patient, or they may meet someone in a support group or hospital setting. Most of the time, the other families are happy to share their stories and offer support to someone else going through the same ordeal. For the child, seeing someone who's actually been through it all and is doing well can be a real boost.

One of the most difficult choices that a parent or patient will have to make is deciding when to stop treatment. Despite the best efforts of everyone involved, there are times that the cancer just does not respond to treatment. Doctors may begin to recommend more experimental treatments to give the child a chance at survival. These experimental treatments are not for everyone, though, and the family needs to decide how aggressively they want the child treated under these circumstances. These experimental therapies may be at different stages of use—they may or may not work in the patient's type of cancer. Often, the experimental treatments are offered only at select centers across the country, so getting to one of them may mean taking the child to a different state just to be treated. This can be even more disruptive to other family members, such as siblings, than the regular therapy was. Reasons for pursuing an experimental treatment include: offering the child a "last chance" at a cure, or helping other children who get this type of cancer in the future to have a better chance at survival. Whatever the reason, this is one decision that no parent ever wants to be forced to make for his or her child.

In general, the choices that parents and patients face are often the same choices that others have faced in the past. Using available resources, such as physicians, nurses, other patients, other families, and written information about the subject, can aid in the decision-making process. Families should be aggressive in seeking these resources and not afraid to ask others for help.

# Chapter 15

## UNDERSTANDING THE MEDICAL SYSTEM

For people who have little experience dealing with the medical system, having a child diagnosed with cancer opens up a new and complicated world. This is especially true for inpatients who spend days and nights, sometimes even weeks at a time, in the hospital setting.

### THE HIERARCHY OF PHYSICIANS

Parents and patients meet many, many people during their hospitalizations. It is nearly impossible to keep the names and faces straight during a time that is filled with uncertainty and fear. Who do you trust? Who is in charge? Wading through the hierarchy of white coats can be difficult and frustrating for many people. In most cases, when a child is undergoing treatment for cancer, he is getting this treatment in a major medical facility. These major medical centers are more often than not teaching hospitals. At a teaching hospital, a patient can expect to be seen by many different stages of "doctors in training" during his hospital stay.

At the bottom of the training ladder is the medical student. Medical students are people who have graduated from college and are undergoing post-graduate studies in medicine with the goal of becoming a licensed physician. Medical school is usually completed in four years, and most of the time, when a medical student is seeing patients in the hospital she is already into her third or fourth year of training. These students may or may not introduce themselves as doctors. They are often wearing the short white coat that goes just past the waist. Medical students cannot write orders for patients without a physician checking and signing off on it. While it can be frustrating at times to deal with someone so junior, medical students are sometimes very helpful, because they are very interested in collecting information. They may ask a detailed question that no one else asks, and that information could be a key in deciding treatment (even if they don't always realize it). The difficulty comes in pulling that information back out of the student in a way that is useful to the other treating providers.

The next step up is the intern. Interns are usually in their first year of practice after completing medical school. Medical students apply for internships at various programs across the country and are accepted on a competitive basis. They are true physicians and are allowed to call themselves "doctor," but they usually are not yet licensed in their field. Interns may or may not be working in the medical specialty they are planning to practice for the rest of their lives. For example, someone who wants to become a radiologist often has to do rotations (often month-long blocks) in different areas of medicine before he can start his training in radiology. A child with cancer will mostly encounter interns that are in the field of pediatrics; these doctors want to work with children, and are typically well-suited for caring for children.

After the year of internship is complete, interns become residents. Residents can be junior or senior, depending on how far away from internship they are. Most residencies in the United States last anywhere from three to six years (including the year of internship). Most pediatrics residencies last three or four years. Typically, the more senior the resident, the more experienced he is, and he should at this stage be able to care for children with serious illness. Both residents and interns are able to write orders regarding patient care, usually without a supervisor. Many residents are also licensed physicians.

Once residency is over, these individuals can practice as autonomous pediatricians in the general workforce. They are able to take board certifications in the field of pediatrics, and they can see patients as they choose. However, many graduates of pediatric residency programs wish to become specialists in one particular field of pediatric medicine, such as neurology or oncology. To become a pediatric subspecialist, residents will apply for fellowship programs that offer them this specialized training. These programs are somewhat more competitive than internships and residencies, and fewer numbers of people are accepted into these programs.

The pediatric oncology fellowship lasts three years. These fellows are often licensed, board-certified pediatricians, who are now pursuing a career in pediatric oncology. The fellowship involves not only patient care, but research as well. Many centers treating patients with cancer do not have fellowship programs, so many patients and families will never encounter a fellow. Fellows are the primary oncology providers for many patients with pediatric cancer, and they work hand in hand with senior oncologists in deciding care.

After the fellowship is complete, the doctor is considered an attending physician. The attending is the person in charge of everyone else on the medical team (i.e., the medical student, the intern, the resident, the fellow, and any other ancillary staff that may be involved). For the parent, the attending oncologist (and in some cases the fellow) is the best person to answer difficult questions about care, therapies, and problems in the hospital. However, the attending is in charge of many other patients and may have the least amount of time to spend with any one patient. In pediatric cancer patients, though, the attending understands the severity of the situation and typically is more willing to devote a good portion of her time to each child, helping to ensure that all of the family's questions are adequately answered.

## OTHER MEDICAL TEAM MEMBERS

One of the most noticeable members of the medical care team is the nurse. In pediatric cancer patients, most of the time a registered nurse (RN) is highly involved in patient care. This nurse has received intense training in nursing skills and is often trained separately in cancer patients and chemotherapy administration. The nurse is responsible for administering all medications ordered by the physicians and for taking care of the overall well-being of the patient.

Many institutions have other nurses, often licensed vocational nurses (LVNs), or medical technicians who assist in the care of patients in the hospital. These healthcare providers are often responsible for getting vital signs (blood pressure, heart rate, temperature, etc.) of the patients at routine intervals throughout the day. They also may have other patient care duties assigned to them, depending on their skill level and comfort with patient care.

In some of the larger medical centers, nurse practitioners will care for patients. These providers have done extended training after obtaining their nursing license (generally a master's degree), which has prepared them for more extensive patient care and has given them greater diagnostic skills than an RN. In some states, nurse practitioners are able to write prescriptions or orders for patients, just as a physician can. In the field of pediatric oncology, the nurse practitioners are often wonderful assets to the treatment team. They can provide excellent care to oncology patients, and they are often knowledgeable enough about the treatment plans to answer any questions posed by the patients or their parents.

Other hospital professionals patients may see during their hospital stay include respiratory therapists (providers who administer breathing treatments and chest physiotherapy), phlebotomists (providers who specialize in blood draws), radiology technicians, child life specialists (providers who work in educating children about their illness through age-appropriate activities), and social workers.

## AN INPATIENT IN A TEACHING HOSPITAL

It can be extremely difficult to adjust to life in a hospital setting. Parents and patients are plagued with poor sleep, many interruptions, early morning rounds, and tests of all types. A stay in the hospital can be absolutely miserable for many. It may be helpful to understand why certain things are done in this way.

For many people, morning rounds are not pleasant. Often, one or many people (usually medical students, interns, or residents) will enter the room sometime before sunrise to ask you questions about the previous night and to perform some semblance of a physical examination. Doctors know that most people would rather sleep during this time, but in order to be effective in delivering patient care, they have to start work very early in the morning. In a teaching hospital, many of the students, interns, and residents have to participate in organized teaching sessions that usually are scheduled around seven or eight o'clock in the morning. After these sessions are complete, they are expected to be able to discuss the patient's active medical issues with the fellow or attending physician in rounds. If the junior people haven't examined the patient and collected the data early enough, they will not have time to prepare for the questions that the senior physicians will ask them. During these rounds, plans will be made for each patient's care during the day. Medications and tests will be ordered and consultations with other services may be placed. The process of rounds can take several hours on very busy patient care services.

At some point after rounds (and in some cases during rounds), the attending physician will try to visit with the patients and their families. The timing of this visit may change depending on any other duties and responsibilities the attending has for the day. Sometimes the attending gets useful information from the patient at this visit that wasn't available earlier (it helps to be awake), and this information can often change the care plan for the patient.

Later in the day, the medical care team begins to collect the data and information from the tests that were ordered, and often this information is shared with the patient and parents. Some families may feel neglected by the medical care team, because they don't get to see the doctors enough during the day. If this is the case, parents should have the nurse ask the doctor to come talk with them when possible. This request may not be answered immediately, but in most cases the doctor will happily come back to the room to discuss care plans with the family.

Consultant physicians (doctors from other specialty services such as gastroenterology or infectious disease) may arrive in the room at any time during the day. Since they are only consulting on the patient and they are not responsible for the daily care, they tend to come around later in the day than the other teams. It is important to remember that the attending oncology physician is still the person in charge of the patient, and sometimes the oncologist will disagree with recommendations made by these consultants.

For many children, the afternoon is their quiet time away from the doctors. For others, this can still be a very busy time of the day for various reasons. Some patients will be getting radiology or blood tests done during this time. Others will be doing schoolwork. Of course, many patients just need their rest to help cope with their illness.

In the early evening hours, the daytime physician team will prepare to leave and the night team will take over the care of the patients. This "on-call" team is usually quite familiar with the patients that they are caring for, but sometimes they may not be familiar with all the intricacies of the child's care. The physicians who actually stay in the hospital overnight are usually interns and residents. There will be a few attending physicians in key areas of the hospital, such as the emergency room or intensive care units, if an emergency occurs. Otherwise, the oncology attendings usually "take call" from home, and the doctors in the hospital will page them if they have any questions about the patients. If a serious problem occurs, the attending may return to the hospital to help with the care in person.

Sometimes the on-call team will do their own rounds on the patients, making sure that everyone is taken care of. However, there are usually fewer total doctors in the hospital at night and often the same amount of work to do as there was during the day, so these doctors are kept quite busy dealing with priority issues. Few patient tests occur in the middle of the night, but this doesn't always mean that the patient is allowed to sleep without interruption. Medications still have to be given and nurses and technicians need to ensure that the patient is not having any complications.

The nurses and technicians are often the lifeline for pediatric patients and their families. Having a caring, knowledgeable nurse can make all the difference during a difficult hospitalization. Most patients see the nurse more often than any other healthcare provider during the day and night, because that nurse is responsible for medications, fluids, food, and many other details of the hospital care. The nurse is usually one of the first to find out if the patient is having a particular problem. Then, the nurse will inform the doctor (usually an intern or resident), who will come and evaluate the situation. The nurse is also often responsible for following up on any changes that happen with the patient's status or care. Nurses typically work in shifts; these shifts are often 12 hours long, and during that shift they are moving constantly, caring for a handful of assigned patients. Many nurses will develop a close relationship with certain oncology patients and their families, and they may try to be assigned certain patients during their scheduled shifts.

## LIFE IN THE CLINIC/OUTPATIENT VISITS

Many childhood cancer patients receive the majority of their care as an outpatient, or in the clinic setting. The physician hierarchy system remains the same, whether the patient is an inpatient or an outpatient, but the patient and family interactions with the medical system may be quite different.

The majority of pediatric oncology centers across the United States use a "team" approach when caring for patients. Once a child is diagnosed with cancer, they typically start getting their care under a specific attending oncologist, who will remain their primary oncologist throughout the treatment course. The attending oncologist likely works with a team of other health care providers, such as an oncology fellow, a nurse practitioner, a registered nurse, and a technician. This team also may work closely with a specific social worker or child life specialist. The oncology care team can be beneficial in the case of small children, because it helps children develop a sense of security by seeing the same providers at each visit. It decreases a lot of the stranger anxiety that children will feel in the clinic setting, and it helps the child feel more comfortable with the surroundings.

Most clinics operate on the same principles: get the patient checked in, take his vital signs (temperature, blood pressure, pulse), get his weight and/ or height, obtain any necessary laboratory studies, and see the nurse assigned to the patient's team. After the nurse has done an initial assessment, the child is seen by a doctor or nurse practitioner on the team. Sometimes, patients will be seen by residents or interns who happen to be working the oncology clinic before seeing one of their usual team members. In other instances, certain members of the treatment team may be absent from the clinic, so the patient is seen by a provider who is covering clinic for them. With time, though, most patients and parents are familiar with nearly all of the healthcare providers who work in the outpatient oncology clinic.

There has been a push in recent years to provide as much treatment as possible in the outpatient setting, rather than bringing the patient into the hospital overnight. Many clinics have special chemotherapy infusion areas where the children come to the clinic just to get the medications. These visits can last several hours, and often the children have to return the next day for the next medication dose. While the child may not be seen by a physician during the chemotherapy infusion visits, there is always a physician nearby in case of problems or questions.

## THE EMERGENCY ROOM

Most families dealing with a child with cancer have experienced the emergency room at some point during her treatment. For many families, the trip to the emergency room (ER) happens in the middle of the night, when the child develops a fever or some bad effect from her cancer. Some ERs have wonderful systems in place for children battling cancer. Others just aren't equipped to handle the care of a child in this special circumstance.

When a child starts treatment for cancer, the pediatric oncologist will discuss all of the "after hours" care options with the family. This usually involves the family contacting the doctor when the problem starts. The oncologist will then instruct the family where to take the child for care. Often, the oncologist will contact the ER as well, giving them notice of the upcoming patient arrival. The oncologist will also try to give the ER instructions on what should be done for the child once they arrive, such as special blood tests, antibiotics, and any extra tests. This process works best when the oncologist and the patient are familiar with the particular ER and when the ER has experience handling children with cancer.

Unfortunately, this process doesn't always work very smoothly. The patient and the family may be out of town visiting relatives when the emergency arises. This may mean going to an unfamiliar ER that may have little or no experience taking care of children in this situation. Some emergency rooms don't have the proper equipment available to access a child's portacath. Others may not understand that a fever in a child with cancer is a true emergency and must be acted on within a short period of time.

Parents need to be prepared for these emergencies, working with the patient's oncologist and the local ER to make sure that the child gets the best care possible. Most families will have some sort of letter stating the child's medical condition, including the cancer diagnosis, current treatment plan, and instructions in case of fever. If the family doesn't have the letter with them, they should have the oncologist talk with the ER directly to give instructions on care.

Sometimes, the ER has its own protocol in place for dealing with children, and this may go against the standard of care for children with cancer. One common concern is the use of rectal thermometers. Many ERs use rectal thermometers to get accurate temperature readings in children. However, an oncology patient who is at risk for low blood counts should almost *never* have a rectal temperature taken, because it puts the child at risk for trauma to the anal area and subsequent infection or abscess in that region. Some parents have had to physically block their child from well-meaning ER staff to prevent them from performing rectal temperatures on the patient.

Caregivers should also have an "emergency kit" for the emergency room. This kit should include numbing cream to put over the port, extra port access needles, information about the patient's medical history (including contact information for the child's pediatric oncologist), a set of overnight items and/or clothes, and perhaps some snacks. It is helpful to keep these items in a bag, ready to go at a moment's notice, because it always seems that the emergency situations happen at the worst possible times.

## WHO CAN WE TRUST?

The patient's attending oncology physician is the person that should have the last say in the child's cancer care. Most patients and families develop a special relationship with this doctor from the beginning of treatment. If there are discrepancies in information relayed to the family by various healthcare providers, the attending is the person making the final decision. However, many members of the oncology care team may be just as knowledgeable about the treatment plan and may be more readily accessible than the attending physician. Families quickly learn who they feel comfortable with and who they can trust for information.

In some circumstances, patients and their families may think that they're not being given the whole story about the cancer or its treatment. When doubt creeps into this relationship, it can cause significant problems for the child's care. Most attending physicians want to know if the family is distrustful of information or unhappy with the care of their child. Pediatric oncologists in particular are very sensitive to these concerns and will usually go out of their way to make sure that the family is comfortable and confident about the care that their child is receiving.

Second opinions in the field of pediatric oncology are not unexpected. With life and death illnesses such as cancer, parents want only the best for their child, and pediatric oncologists are usually willing to obtain second opinions for difficult cases. The national community of pediatric oncologists is small; these physicians will often contact other oncologists at institutions all across the country if they think that another opinion will aid in the care of a child with cancer. If the pediatric oncology attending is unwilling to listen to the family's concerns about the diagnosis or care of their child, the family will lose faith in the physician and the medical care system, and the child's cancer treatment will suffer.

# Chapter 16

⤜ˢ

# UNDERSTANDING
# CLINICAL TRIALS

⤜ˢ

When a person is diagnosed with cancer in the United States, they are often asked to participate in research. This is especially true for children and adolescents with cancer. This section discusses the reasons why young cancer patients are often the subject of research studies.

## WHY RESEARCH?

Pediatric cancer treatment is a real success story in terms of improvement in survival rates and outcomes. Children who were diagnosed with some form of cancer in the early 1950s were often sent home to die. Less than 10 percent of these children were expected to survive their disease, because there were few effective treatment options, and the disease was so rare that no one person had enough experience to come up with a strong treatment plan. Fortunately, because it was such a rare disease, physicians started coming together as groups to help figure out these devastating diseases and to come up with effective treatment plans. In the late 1950s, a handful of institutions joined together through the National Cancer Institute to work on research studies in children with leukemia. Through their work, chemotherapy was shown to be an effective treatment in many patients with childhood leukemia.

Since leukemia therapy was progressing, similar treatment trials were started for young patients with solid tumors. Treatment included many different therapy groups, such as surgery, radiation, and chemotherapy. This led to groups of physicians from different specialties of medicine, all with one common goal—to cure children with cancer. The National Cancer Institute physician groups began to grow, and eventually these treatment studies were spread throughout the country. In the 1980s, the cure rates for childhood cancer had increased to 50 percent, and today, survival rates approach 80 percent.

The basic concept behind pediatric cancer research is comparing two or more treatment plans with each other, based on how they actually work in children battling cancer. One treatment plan usually has the designation of "standard of care," which means that it is the best known treatment for the disease. The other treatment is different, but has real potential for benefiting the child receiving the new therapy. Until the newer therapy has been shown to be better than the previous standard treatment, the new therapy is often considered experimental. Many times, these newer treatment plans offer a significant benefit to the patient, but sometimes the standard treatment is better.

In some cancer subtypes, the number of patients who develop the disease in a set period of time is so low that direct comparison of the different types of treatment is difficult. In these cases, only the new treatment is studied, and the results are compared to historical survival rates for the disease (taken from the best known treatment available before the new study was started). Others, such as many types of leukemia, have enough new patients diagnosed each year that two or more treatments are compared head to head at the same time in the same research study to see which has the better outcome.

Looking at which treatment is best is not the only kind of research done in pediatric cancer patients. Other research involves looking for signs that certain patients are more likely to do better or worse than other patients. This can be through various genetic tests on the cancer cells, or through different factors related to the location of the disease, the age of the patient, or the way the cancer cells act. Many research studies in pediatric cancer involve "banking" tumor tissue; physicians will ask parents or patients to agree that a small amount of the cancer specimen will be deposited into a tissue bank, where studies may be run on the tumor tissue at a later time. These future studies could include analysis of potential new cancer treatments on specific cancer cells. There is another type of research done in pediatric cancer patients that looks at trends in different types of cancer. This epidemiology (study of the population) research often involves getting information about the cancer diagnosis for a cancer registry. Collected information often includes the age of the patient, the type of cancer, how far the cancer has spread, and how the child does with treatment. This information can be extremely helpful for future plans in cancer treatment and research.

## SHOULD I ALLOW MY CHILD TO BE TREATED IN A RESEARCH STUDY?

*I remember sitting in Michael's hospital room, still in shock about being told just a few hours ago that he had leukemia. Then, a doctor came into the room talking to me about a research study for children with leukemia. Research? I couldn't believe that she had the nerve to suggest that I let Michael be treated like a guinea pig on some research study. He deserved the best treatment possible—how could making him a test case give him the best treatment? [Excerpt from a conversation with a mother of a child with leukemia.]*

Many parents are put off by physicians wanting to enter their child into a research study. The thought of research may conjure up images of lab rats getting injections or mad scientists working on strange experiments. It is hard enough to accept that a child has cancer, and the thought of putting them through some experimental treatment is terrifying for most people. However, most parents and patients will be approached by someone soon after the diagnosis to see if they will allow the child to be placed on a treatment protocol, which is the formal term for the research study being offered.

As difficult as is sounds, there are many cases in which research treatments really do offer the child the best treatment. In general, children who receive a cancer treatment while on a research study do better than other children who receive the exact same cancer treatment without the research study. This is potentially related to the specific guidelines that physicians must follow when treating a patient on a strict treatment plan. Individual physicians treating a patient may take more liberties in the therapy than would a group of physicians treating patients per a research study. Another benefit for many patients on research studies is the automatic "second opinion" that they receive on the pathology report. Most pediatric cancer research protocols have a group of pathology specialists who re-examine each patient's tumor to confirm the exact diagnosis.

Some individual hospitals have their own pediatric cancer research studies, but the majority of pediatric cancer treatment centers in North America (and even a few internationally) are members of the Children's Oncology Group, or COG. This group of over 250 medical institutions is supported by the National Cancer Institute (NCI). COG was formed in 2000 with the merger of several other national organizations involved in treating childhood cancer. Individual hospitals must meet strict criteria to be members of COG, and treatment recommended by COG is considered the standard of care therapy by most physicians and insurance companies in the United States.

Being part of a national standard of care treatment plan can be comforting to many parents facing a new diagnosis of cancer. Sometimes people assume that only the "big name" centers can take good care of children with cancer, but traveling to these centers for treatment often only adds to the family stress, because the home support system is lost. Any institution that is a member of COG can offer excellent care to children with cancer, and likely, the treatment plan used in Nebraska is the same as the one used in New York, or Texas, or California. Children in general are able to get the best possible treatment for their cancer at any of these locations. Occasionally, a specific type of cancer may require specialized therapy that is not available at a particular institution, such as proton radiation therapy. In these instances, children may receive part of their treatment in one location and the rest of the treatment in another. Parents and patients have to trust that the child's oncologist is looking out for the child's best interests.

*After I listened to Michael's doctor about the reason for the research study and the potential benefit for him and the many children out there who may get leukemia in the future, I started to understand why the research was necessary. But I was still uncomfortable about him being a guinea pig. The doctor left me a lot of information about the research study—too much to digest in a short period of time. She told me to think about Michael and the way I wanted him to be treated. She wanted me to discuss the research plan with friends and family members so I could get other opinions on his treatment. I wrote down several questions that came up during my reading and family discussions. When she returned the next morning, we talked more about this whole research thing and she seemed to answer all of my questions honestly. I finally decided to go with the research treatment plan, so she asked me to sign a consent form allowing him to be treated on the study. The consent form was very long, but she went over it with me in detail until I was more comfortable with what I was signing. I felt reassured that we could take him off the study at any time if I had any doubts or second thoughts.*

*I didn't have a lot of time to consider other options because Michael needed to start treatment as soon as possible, but I also didn't feel rushed by the process. Never rush into a treatment that you're not informed about unless your child is so emergently sick that you have no choice. I've noticed that most of Michael's doctors want me to understand everything I can about his medicines and his treatment plan, and they always encourage me to ask questions if I have concerns. [Excerpt from a conversation with a mother of a child with leukemia.]*

# PARTICIPATION IN CLINICAL TRIALS

The research studies used in pediatric cancer therapy are also known as clinical trials. While pediatric oncologists often like to treat children on these research protocols, sometimes there are no trials available for patients with certain diagnoses. These trials are open for set periods of time, and sometimes a patient gets diagnosed with a disease during a period that is "in between" trials.

All clinical research studies have criteria that patients must meet to be eligible for the treatment. These are called inclusion criteria, and they include things like age, the subtype of cancer, and previous treatment history. Some things about patients make them ineligible for a study. These are called exclusion criteria, and often include things like pregnancy, problems with the liver, or other illnesses or conditions that may be present at the start of treatment.

Any treatment given to a patient for any type of disease comes with risks. Many cancer treatments have higher risks than the treatments used for other diseases. This often translates to greater risk with medications or therapies that may be considered "experimental." When creating these trials, investigators try to weigh the risks and benefits of each individual treatment before considering the treatment for any patient.

There are specific rules that must be followed for a clinical trial. There are outside groups that review these studies to ensure that patients are being treated fairly and ethically. COG clinical trials must be approved by a national review board prior to being allowed to enroll any patients. Many hospitals also conduct their own separate review of any research being done in their facility to ensure patient safety and confidentiality. This review is usually done by an Institutional Review Board (IRB), which is an independent committee made up of health care providers, community members, statisticians, and other groups. The IRB ensures that the proposed trial will protect the participants and that patients will be treated ethically. In COG trials, there is no reimbursement given to individuals who participate in the studies, and typically there is no extra cost for the treatments proposed, outside of the usual insurance co-payments and treatment costs.

# DIFFERENT PHASES OF CLINICAL TRIALS

When different treatment plans are used on a clinical trial in pediatric cancer therapy, they go through different phases of study. Each "phase" of the trial has a different purpose in studying an experimental drug or therapy plan. The lower the phase, the less information participants are given about the treatment. Before studies are conducted on people, the medicines are tested in a laboratory setting, either on small clusters of cancer cells or in animal subjects. If a treatment is promising in this setting, it may then be approved for use in clinical trials.

Phase I trials are small trials, usually conducted only at a few select places, involving a small number of people (often less than 30). The purpose of a phase I trial is to get an assessment of how well the treatment is tolerated, how safe it is, and how the treatment should be delivered in the body. In cancer patients, these trials are typically done on those who have no other good treatment options available. These patients may have exhausted all other known effective treatment for their disease, and it is usually expected they will not survive their cancer. Phase I trial treatments are not done in these people to cure them of their cancer; they are conducted to see if the medicine can be tolerated in others. On rare occasions, the medicine given in a phase I trial does help the patient and successfully treats his cancer.

Often in pediatric cancer phase I studies, the investigator is trying to determine the highest dose of the medicine that can be given a person without causing that person significant harm. For instance, the first three patients enrolled may be given a very low dose. If they don't have bad side effects, then the next three patients will get a slightly higher dose. If those three don't have bad side effects, then the next three patients will get an even higher dose. This escalation of dosage continues until patients start to have problems with the medication. The information about what dose is more easily tolerated gives information for the next phase of study.

Phase II trials begin with a treatment that has been shown to be safe at the dose prescribed by the phase I study. These studies are larger that phase I studies and are run on more patients in more treatment centers. Phase II trials are done with the purpose of seeing if a medicine works in the disease being treated. By testing higher numbers of patients, sometimes phase II trials pick up unexpected but important side effects that were not seen in the smaller number of patients studied in the phase I trial.

Phase III trials are the most common trials conducted in patients with pediatric cancer. Here, the patient is treated with a therapy that should work (as shown by information obtained in a phase II study), and often this newer therapy is compared to the best known treatment available. To compare these different types of treatment, patients are often "randomized" to one treatment plan or another. This randomization is usually computer-generated, but in essence is like flipping a coin, with each patient having an equal chance of getting one or the other type of treatment.

# KEY THINGS TO REMEMBER ABOUT RESEARCH

While many people choose to allow their children to be a part of one or more research studies during their treatment for cancer, no one is ever forced to take this path. If a family is feeling too much pressure from the physician about participating in a research study, they should let the physician know. Often, the oncologist is very passionate about research and knows how it has helped many children with cancer survive their disease. However, in most instances, the oncologist does not want to pressure anyone into enrolling in a study, and there are times when the oncologist may even discourage enrollment if the treatment is not right for the individual patient.

Parents should feel that they have adequate time to digest the information presented to them. The physician and the parents should discuss the consent forms and treatment at length prior to anything being signed. Patients who are seven years old or older should also have a chance to discuss the treatment plans with their parents and doctor. Most oncologists will ask the child also to sign the consent form in assent of the treatment. This gives the patient more of a feeling of control about what she will be facing in the upcoming months. There are instances where teenagers under the age of 18 will disagree with the treatment plan and refuse to sign the assent. If this happens, the child or teenager should not be enrolled on the research treatment. This does not, however, mean that they will not be treated, and the physicians and parents will come to an agreement about what is the best treatment for the patient.

Parents and patients may take themselves off of the study plan at any time. This process should be easy to do and should be explained by the provider prior to signing any consent for therapy. Again, not being treated per the study does not mean that no treatment will be given. The physicians will work with the family and the patient to determine the best available therapy for the cancer.

Sometimes research studies have nothing to do with treating the patient's cancer. There are studies that center on things like quality of life for the patient or long-term effects of therapy. They may involve a questionnaire or intelligence testing. While these things may seem fairly innocuous, the same information and consent process will be conducted for these non-treatment studies as well, with the same patient protections in place.

# Chapter 17

⤳

# ASKING QUESTIONS, FINDING ANSWERS

⤳

After a serious illness hits a family, many people start to ask why. "Why me? Why my child? What did we do to deserve this?" There is almost never a satisfactory answer to the question, "Why?"

*When Andrew was diagnosed with his brain tumor, I was stunned. How could a FOUR-year-old deserve to get a brain tumor? He had never done anything bad to anyone. He was a sweet, innocent child with his whole life ahead of him— why did he have to get cancer? His mother and I actually had someone come up to us and tell us that we must have done something wrong to make this happen. That this was just "payback" for something horrible in our past, and now it was affecting our child. Of course, we didn't believe them, but hearing that come out of someone else's mouth was really painful. At the time, neither one of us knew how to react. [Excerpt from a conversation with a father of a child with an ependymoma.]*

While most parents don't get told outright that they are to blame for their child's cancer diagnosis, there are many parents who feel responsible for what is happening to their child. Many things are running through the mind of a parent whose child has just been diagnosed with cancer, and guilty thoughts are often present.

Some parents wonder if their child wouldn't have cancer if they brought them in for care sooner. Parents need to realize, though, that even if they had sought medical care earlier, their child would still end up with the diagnosis of cancer. Many people will examine previous experiences or exposures that could be related to cancer. Some mothers go back to the time of pregnancy or even conception, trying to come up with something that made this cancer happen. There are very few instances in pediatric cancer where a true cause is found for the child later developing his or her disease.

Siblings may handle the diagnosis of cancer differently. Some brothers and sisters feel that *they* are being punished for something they've done to the cancer patient. They may recall an argument that they had; maybe some hurtful things were said, and now they are afraid that the sick child is going to die. Others become very resentful of the child who has cancer. While they understand that cancer is a serious illness, the siblings may feel that cancer is punishing them because they no longer get attention from their parents, other family members, or friends. The sick child gets the majority of attention, and the sibling can become quite jealous of the situation.

Older children and adolescents often blame themselves for their cancer diagnosis. They may feel that they have cancer because they need to be punished for something that they did. Not only do they have an illness that may cause physical pain and suffering, but they may also become more isolated from friends and can't participate in their usual activities. It can be extremely difficult to get out of this cycle of illness, disappointment, and pain. However, once teenagers are able to get past the initial diagnosis, they are often the patients best equipped to help others deal with their own illnesses.

In general, it is important to know that there is no one reason why anyone gets cancer. No one individual is responsible for the diagnosis, and there is no one to blame for the disease. Directing the anger and frustration directly at the cancer can be helpful in the fight against it and can empower the patient through her medical treatments.

## THE "NORMAL" LIFE WITH CANCER

The concept of a "normal" life during cancer treatment is very foreign to many individuals. How can a family lead a normal life when everything has been turned upside down by this disease? The truth is that life changes, sometimes dramatically, after cancer hits a child, but there can be a new "normal" in the lives of patients and family members dealing with those changes.

Consistency is important for families fighting cancer. While it may not be possible to be consistent in all of the daily routines, parents and patients can find some consistency in certain areas of their life. Trying to keep children in school whenever possible allows them to stay connected to friends, classmates, and teachers who were important parts of their lives before the cancer diagnosis. For children who can't physically attend school, keeping up with schoolwork and learning can be important in helping with a sense of normalcy. Many children were active in sports prior to being diagnosed with cancer, and keeping them on their sports teams can be a great outlet for their emotions. Even if they aren't capable of playing in the soccer game or swimming at a meet, they can get a much-needed boost from their teammates by just suiting up and attending.

Some children will focus on food during their treatments. Cancer treatments may alter a child's taste buds, but there may be particular food items that bring them a sense of comfort. While it is unreasonable to expect extravagant home-cooked meals all the time, it may be possible to keep up with some of the child's favorite foods on a mealtime schedule similar to that used before the diagnosis.

Others need an outlet for their feelings about their diagnosis. For some, this comes with drawing; for others, writing or music. Providing a child the means to tell his story can help him feel like he has a purpose with his illness. Also, allowing a cancer patient to participate in his own care gives him a sense of control. It is important to let the child discuss things about his treatments that are bothering him and to let him have a say in the way things are done.

The subject of discipline for a child with cancer is difficult to handle. Many parents and family members feel so sorry for the sick child that they want to let her do whatever she wants. Giving in to all the desires of a child can lead to significant problems down the road, and contrary to belief, it often does not make the child any happier.

> *I knew that I was really sick when I started getting all these presents. People gave me so many stuffed animals, toys, and video games that I couldn't even fit them all in my hospital room. When I got home, my parents let me eat whatever I wanted to eat and go to bed whenever I wanted to. I didn't have to do any chores anymore, and my sister was really mad at me for that. I started to think that I must be going to die, because I could do anything I wanted to. My parents didn't treat me the same way anymore, and I missed that. [Excerpt from a conversation with a child with Ewing's sarcoma.]*

When a child is spoiled early on in therapy, they often become difficult to manage later on during the treatment. Parents become very frustrated trying to care for a child who thinks only of himself, and behaviors only get worse as the therapy continues. Behavior problems often persist after treatment is over. Many childhood cancer survivors have significant problems with reckless behaviors when they get older, sometimes related to a lack of limitations during their treatment.

Many families have to face difficult issues when trying to help their child lead a normal life during treatment. For instance, if a child has a brain tumor and has to undergo surgery as part of the treatment, that child may have significant neurological deficits present after the surgery. Another example would be a child undergoing treatment for cancer who gets a serious infection that affects her body's function and leads to brain damage. Some children require life-altering surgery, such as amputation, to treat their cancer. All of these extreme treatment instances require special help in getting life back to "normal."

Every child who suffers through cancer treatment is different, and each child will have his own set of issues to deal with. How do you convince a soccer star who lost part of her leg that she can play soccer again? How do you explain to a teenager with a brain tumor that he may have to re-learn many of the things he used to be able to do, such as talking, writing, or walking? How can you reconcile the image of the child before her cancer diagnosis with the image of a child who is tired, sick, bald, and miserable?

There are no great answers to any of these questions, and healthcare providers may not be able to help out in ways that they would like to. Often, parents are left to their own devices; they have to come up with some method to handle the tremendous changes that have occurred in their lives, and many of these changes have unimaginable consequences. Talking with other families going through similar situations can be extremely helpful. Getting information about the cancer itself and its treatments can also give some clues as to how to deal with the changes. Using psychologists who have a special interest or training in the field of childhood cancer can be extremely helpful for families in difficult situations.

## THE FUTURE AFTER CANCER

Once cancer has struck a child, the effects of the illness often last a lifetime. There are potential emotional, educational, and physical concerns that can hang over these families indefinitely. Patients and their families have to deal with the emotional distress related to the diagnosis and the potential that the disease could return. There are often physical concerns related to the treatments for the cancer that may linger in patients, preventing them from doing certain activities that they used to love. Others have difficulties achieving the educational and vocational goals they had laid out for themselves before the diagnosis.

After families are able to get past the initial shock of the cancer diagnosis, their attentions may shift to the future. Will my son get his football scholarship? Will my daughter be able to attend college? Will I ever be a grandparent? Issues surrounding each individual child play a part in determining his future.

> *We found out Sharonda had a brain tumor when she was 14 years old. She had surgery to take out the tumor, and then she had to get radiation treatments. She was so tired all the time, and after the surgery she had a hard time using her right arm. She wasn't able to go to school, and she couldn't hang out with her friends. Sharonda loved dancing and had hoped to attend a major dance school over the summer, but after she got cancer she just didn't think it could happen. I hated seeing her so sad—it was like she had given up on her dreams and she didn't even want to think about the future.*
>
> *A few months after she finished her radiation treatments, she started to get her energy level back. Once she had more energy, she started up with her dancing again. It was tough—she had to do a lot of "catch-up" work, and her arm really gave her a lot of problems with the dance moves. Thankfully, she was able to continue dancing, and two years after finding out she had the brain tumor, she finally got to spend her summer at dance school. That was a turning point for her, because she knew that if she worked hard enough, her dreams could still come true. [Excerpt from a conversation of a mother of a child with an astrocytoma.]*

In general, schools will try to work with families and children who are dealing with major medical problems. Some schools and school systems are more understanding than others, but usually some sort of compromise can be worked out. Many children undergo neuropsychiatric testing (similar to IQ testing) after they have finished their cancer treatment. This testing can help educators determine which method of learning works best for the child. By making special accommodations for students who have specific problems with reading comprehension or excessive school work loads (related to their cancer treatment), these children can still excel in school and achieve their goals.

Sometimes children and families have to adjust their view of the future. There are instances when the cancer and its treatments lead to long-term functional problems that keep the child from ever living a truly independent life, requiring more long-term support. For many, this transition from the happy, healthy, "normal" child to one who will have chronic handicaps can be devastating, and it brings its own set of grief issues.

Another concern for parents of children with cancer is making the transition to being parents of adults who used to have cancer. The natural instinct to protect your child goes into overdrive for many families who get through treatments for this disease, and it can be very difficult for parents to let go when the time comes. Children and parents both will do better with this transition period if the caregivers instill a sense of independence in the child throughout the course of diagnosis and treatment. This independence can come from something as simple as giving the patient specific responsibilities during treatment—when the child knows that there are specific jobs that need to be done under adult supervision, she is much better prepared for the future when she will have to be responsible for her own care.

# Chapter 18

## HELPING FAMILY MEMBERS AND FRIENDS

When a child is diagnosed with cancer, it can be extremely difficult for the child and other family members to cope with the diagnosis. Once the parent has gotten past letting the child know that he has cancer, the parent is faced with making sure that the child handles the illness in the best way possible. The child's mental attitude about the things going on around him can mean a great deal in the child's fight against cancer. The child's attitude is sometimes a reflection of the parent's attitude, and it is very easy for the parent to get overwhelmed by all of the issues that come with a cancer diagnosis.

The parent often becomes the gateway for information to other well-meaning family members and friends, and this relay of information can become very difficult and tiring. Some parents are happy to have the extra support, especially from close friends and family members on whom they would call for more "ordinary" troubles. However, when something like cancer happens, even those who are mere acquaintances may want to be involved in the day to day aspects of the child's care, and this can be difficult for parents to handle.

There are certain methods that parents can use to help them deal with the flood of support that others want to give. Early on, the parent should designate one family member or close friend to become the new gateway for information. This designee should be responsible for relaying all the information to others about new medical information and updates to the child's care. Sometimes, it may be simpler for the parents to meet with a group of friends or family members and have them disperse the information to others, thus decreasing some of the work for the parents.

Parents need to understand that they don't have to talk to everyone—it is perfectly acceptable to tell others that you are too tired or just can't talk at that time. If necessary, the parent can leave a simple message on the answering machine regarding the situation or giving contact information for another person. Using Caller ID, the parents can screen incoming calls and speak only to the people they are ready to talk to.

Some medical centers allow parents easy access to the Internet. There are specific Web sites available for situations such as this, where the family can create a Web page for the child. This Web page can give information about the diagnosis, hospital address, contact information, and other important details about active issues. The caregivers can update the Web site through journal entries as often as they like, giving others a place to go to get good information about the child's progress. The Web sites also usually have a "guestbook" area, where well-wishers can leave positive thoughts, comments, or greetings to the parents or child. The guestbook postings can be read at the convenience of the caregiver, and they can be a real boost when medical issues aren't going very well.

Many people may want to help, but most don't have any idea what they can do for the family. When time allows, it may be best to come up with a list of specific tasks that need to be completed. These may include meals, shopping, laundry, yard work, babysitting duties for the other children, or pet care. It may be best to keep one close friend or family member in charge of this chore list, so things can be organized and completed appropriately.

## KEEPING SIBLINGS INFORMED AND CARED FOR

Many parents of a child with cancer also have other children under their care. Even under the best of circumstances, the relationships between the parents and the other children can become strained during this difficult time. Parents need to be up-front with siblings, letting them know how sick the patient is, how long he will be in the hospital, and what the treatments are going to entail.

Depending on the age of the sibling, there are some predictable responses and concerns regarding siblings of cancer patients. In many ways, the siblings are "punished" for the patient's cancer in indirect ways. They have to see the emotional stress on their parents and other family members, wondering if they are somehow to blame for the problems. Siblings are faced with more time away from their parents because the sick child needs so much attention. Day-to-day activities such as after-school sports or dance lessons may become uncertain, because they don't know if someone will be able to take them to these events.

Often, siblings feel a sense of guilt about the whole situation. In some cases, the sibling may have been angry with the patient prior to the diagnosis, hoping that something bad would happen to them. Now that something bad has happened, they may feel somewhat responsible. In other instances, siblings feel guilty for being healthy. It may not seem fair that they can be healthy and active while their sick brother or sister is in the hospital all the time, away from friends, school, and home life.

On the other hand, siblings also have a tendency to become jealous at some point during the cancer therapy. In a way, they almost wish that they had cancer too. If they had cancer, they would be getting all the attention. The parents would be spending time with them. Family members and friends would be talking about them. They would be getting presents all the time. They wouldn't be ignored by the doctors and nurses in the hospital who only seem to care about the patient. This jealousy can turn in to anger, resentment, or depression, and it can lead to more problems with interactions between family members. Some siblings start to change their behaviors to get more attention from others. Unfortunately, these changes are usually in the form of "acting out," leading to their getting into trouble and then receiving the attention they crave.

While it may be very hard for a parent to do so, it is extremely important to focus attention on the siblings as well as the patient. The siblings deserve the love and attention of the parents, without interruptions related to the cancer. Parents need to plan special time with each of the siblings one-on-one, making sure that the siblings feel wanted and loved during this hectic time.

Many times, siblings will come with the patient to the hospital or to the doctor's office. Usually, they will get some attention from the medical staff as well, and it may be helpful for them to know the people and locations so they can picture what the patient is going through during treatments. Time in the hospital or clinic can be a special bonding time between the siblings as well, since there's often not a lot of entertainment for someone stuck in the hospital.

The discipline issues that arise for cancer patients are also present in their siblings. Sometimes, siblings may push their limits to see what type of reaction they will get from their parents. The parents need to be consistent with discipline, not ignoring these infractions. This consistency will help the siblings feel a sense of safety and comfort during a time where other things seem to be changing constantly.

School teachers and classmates of siblings may be allies for parents of children with cancer. Sometimes, the parent may not be able to see subtle changes that are occurring in the siblings. In school-aged children, the teacher may spend more time with them during the day than the parents, so it can be helpful to enlist their help in identifying behavioral changes or issues. Parents should keep the teachers informed about changes in the patient's status. This will help the teachers look more closely for changes that occur in the siblings over the time of the treatment course. Teachers may also be able to help arrange counseling sessions through the school to help siblings cope with the patient's disease.

There may be special sibling support groups available through the same support groups for the cancer patients. These sibling groups are nice because the siblings see that they're not alone in dealing with all of these unique issues. Patients get to see other patients in the clinic or the hospital, but siblings of patients sometimes lead a more isolated life, thinking that they're the only ones dealing with these issues.

# Chapter 19

❧

# WHEN CANCER TREATMENTS STOP WORKING

❧

Cancer is responsible for the most disease-related deaths in children in the United States. While survival rates have increased significantly in the last 50 years, death can still be the endpoint of treatment. The most difficult time for a parent in the fight against their child's cancer comes when nothing else can be done to cure the child.

Some children never even make it to the treatment phase of their cancer therapy. There are many instances of children coming to an emergency room with an undiagnosed illness (which later turns out to be some form of cancer) and dying before any sort of significant treatment can even be started. Some children die suddenly of complications from the treatment, such as an overwhelming infection or sudden stroke. The majority of children who die from pediatric cancer, though, die simply from progression of the cancer itself.

When the parents are told that their child's cancer treatment is not working, they may be faced with several decisions. The first decision involves looking for other forms of treatment. They may discuss other treatment options with their child's oncologist, and there may be some reasonably good but unproven therapies available, depending on the child and the type of cancer. The decision to pursue aggressive treatment in the face of little hope of cure should be made with the child. Quantity of life versus quality of life may need to be analyzed. For example, should the goal be to keep the patient alive for a longer period of time, often sacrificing the quality of the remaining time, or should the goal be to keep the patient as comfortable as possible without treatments that have side effects and require frequent hospital trips? Many children and adolescents will tell their parents that they do not want to start another experimental form of therapy or that they are tired of the treatments and just need to stop. Having the patient's agreement, no matter what path is pursued, can mean a lot for those involved.

Once the patient and family have decided to stop pursuing treatment against the cancer, end-of-life care gets introduced to the family. Palliative care is an important step in this process. The goal of palliative care is to ease the suffering of the patient. Some cancer care centers may actually have palliative care teams that specialize in end-of-life care for children. In many instances, pediatric oncologists are important members of these teams because they are forced to deal with childhood death on a fairly regular basis. There are many important goals to palliative care. These include dealing with not only the physical needs of the patient, but also spiritual and emotional needs. For patients who have been part of a treatment team during their active cancer therapy, this same treatment team may play a key role in their palliative care as well.

There are many grades of palliative care for a child who has lost the fight against cancer. Some families may want the patient to get antibiotics to treat infections. Others may desire blood transfusions for patients who have low blood counts. Some children may not be able to sustain their own dietary needs, so families can request that nutritional support be continued for the patient. Each of these treatment measures are medical interventions that affect the natural process of death in an individual. There are also times that families take a "less is more" approach, avoiding any of these medical interventions and allowing the child to die without receiving these life-sustaining treatments. There is no right or wrong method. All may be appropriate, depending on the wishes and desires of the child and the parents.

## TALKING TO THE CHILD

There is no perfect way to tell a child he or she is going to die. Many children who have been fighting the battle against cancer know something about death, often because they know other children in the oncology center who have died from their disease. They may also have some idea of death from family members who have passed away, pets that have died, or famous people in the movies or television who are no longer living. Sometimes children bring up the question to their parents: "Am I going to die?" This question may present itself at different times during treatment for cancer. At the beginning of their diagnosis, the child senses that the parents are worried; maybe the parents are crying a lot. The child may ask this pointed question because she knows she is sick and sees many sad faces around her. Similar things happen when the cancer has stopped responding to therapy. Parents may become quiet or tearful; the attitude of other friends and family members may change. There are many times that children actually feel the end coming near, and they may bring up the subject of death with their family.

When talking to a child about death, it is extremely important to be honest about the situation. A child dealing with cancer deserves to know the truth about what is happening to him. The age of the child will play a role in how the information is handled. A younger child may equate death to a long sleep. Young school-aged children may think that the death is a punishment for something bad that they did in the past. Older children are more concerned about the details of death—what will happen to them, will they be alone, how will the parents handle them being gone. Teenagers often worry about things that they wish they were able to accomplish during life; they feel a special sense of loss, because death is robbing them of their future.

When a child knows he is going to die, he may express certain wishes to his family and friends. He may want to visit a special relative that he misses, or he may want to attend some particular event or celebration. Some want to experience a new adventure, which can be as simple as seeing a particular movie or as challenging as climbing a mountain. If these experiences are important to the child, they become important to the family as well. Many health care teams will work with the family to help make the child's wishes a reality.

On a smaller scale, it is important to allow the child contact with friends and other family members if they want to see other people. It is important to work to make each remaining day as special for the child as possible. The key is to listen to the child, not superimpose other's wishes and needs on the child.

## THE ROLE OF HOSPICE

When many people think of hospice care, they may picture someone being left alone to die. These people may be hesitant to consider such an option for a child dying of cancer, but for many families, hospice is a wonderful option. Hospice is a form of palliative care that is designed specifically for people with a terminal illness. Hospice care can be provided in many different settings, from the child's home to the hospital. Hospice care usually involves a team of health care providers that focus on the needs of the patient, making her final moments as pleasant and comfortable as possible, allowing her to die gracefully. With hospice in place, family members are more able to focus on the child and not worry about details of medical care.

For some, hospice is not acceptable because they feel that by using hospice, they are giving up on their child's cancer fight. Others may be uncomfortable having the child die at home, so they insist on care being given at some other location. It can be difficult for siblings of cancer patients to deal with the idea of death, and sometimes parents want to protect siblings from having their home be associated with the patient's illness and death. There are also instances where it is easier for the family as a unit to spend time with a dying child when the home is the care center, and the siblings and other family members may consider the home a place with an extra special connection to the patient.

Hospice care teams usually consist of several different healthcare providers, including physicians, nurses, and social workers. This team works closely with the patient's primary oncologist to provide the best care possible for the situation. A patient is never kept from the healthcare team that they have worked closely with during their treatment; the child merely has other providers who specialize in these situations.

## DEALING WITH PAIN

A cancer-related death is often quite painful for the child. One of the primary goals of any healthcare provider caring for a dying child is to help treat the child's pain. Treating a child's pain does not usually do anything to prolong the child's life. It merely makes the last moments more comfortable. Often, pain medications include some form of narcotic medication, such as morphine, fentanyl, or dilaudid. These medications can be given by mouth, through the IV, or even by absorption directly into the skin. The way the medicine is administered usually depends on the circumstances surrounding the child.

Some parents are concerned about narcotic addiction. In general, children with cancer will need some form of narcotic pain management during their cancer therapy. When used appropriately, this narcotic use is not habit-forming. In a terminally ill child, narcotics can be extremely helpful for the patient. Many children dealing with pain from their cancer require very high doses of narcotics to keep their pain under control. In a normal individual, these doses could cause a person to stop breathing and die without having some underlying terminal medical disease. However, in a person dealing with extreme pain, these high doses are necessary, because the person and his pain quickly become tolerant to the doses of narcotics being used. These higher doses are not given with the intent to stop a patient's life, but to stop a patient's pain.

Hospice centers and pediatric oncology teams are quite used to using these high doses of medications at the appropriate time in these special patients. Parents don't want to see their child suffer, and they usually accept the pain medicines that are prescribed.

## AFTER THE CHILD IS GONE

Many people who have lost a child to cancer have had a significant amount of "anticipatory grief" time. While this may provide some help with the grieving process, it still doesn't make this horrible time any easier to deal with. In the days immediately following the death of a child, parents and family members may be focused on funeral preparations, notification of friends and family members, and other unexpected problems that may arise. After the initial few days, however, many different emotions can set in for a child's loved ones. These may include numbness, denial, ambivalence, guilt, fear, anger, and depression. It is very difficult to cope with the loss of a child, and each family member will likely handle this loss in a different way. People may also have physical manifestations of their grief, such as sleeplessness, physical pain, shortness of breath, and fatigue. While these physical symptoms have no medical cure, they can significantly impact the day-to-day activities of a person experiencing them.

When a mother and a father handle the death of a child differently, it can add more stress to an already difficult situation. Add sibling emotions to this mix, and families can be devastated, not just by the child's death, but by the aftermath of grief. Keeping open communication between family members and accepting the fact that not everyone handles grief in the same way can help keep a family together.

Some people handle the death of a child by trying to go on with day-to-day activities as if nothing has happened. While this may be easier for some, it is usually not the best way to handle grief, and this approach can actually hurt other loved ones who need to talk about the child. Ignoring grief and its effects on day-to-day life can be harmful and lead to physical problems. While others may not understand exactly what the caregiver is going through, just having a close friend lend an ear can be helpful in dealing with the loss of a child.

Other activities that may help with the transition are memorial services, volunteer work, creating special memory collections about the child, and keeping a journal or writing about feelings that are being experienced. There are several support groups available for helping people deal with the loss of a child. Others prefer individual or group counseling, or support from religious groups or friends.

# CONCLUSION

When a child is diagnosed with cancer, no one can comprehend how different life will become. From the moment the parents hear the word "cancer," nothing in their lives will ever be quite the same. Simple day-to-day activities such as doing laundry and paying the bills can become monumental tasks when trying to juggle caring for a sick child in the hospital and taking care of other family duties.

Many caregivers are forced to quit their jobs, placing a new financial stress on an emotionally devastating situation. There also are many families who become torn apart by the strain that this illness places on relationships; it is not uncommon for parents to become separated or divorced, either during or after the completion of treatments. Siblings may bear resentment towards the child affected by cancer because of the changes cancer brings to their lives as well.

While cancer is the most common cause of disease-related death in people aged 1 to 20 years, at least the survival rates for pediatric cancer continue to increase as researchers seek for innovative ways to treat this horrific disease. Nearly 80 percent of these children and adolescents will win the battle against their cancer. More focus is being given to the concept of "late effects" of cancer therapy, helping to ensure that the patients who win this battle will also be able to enjoy life as happy and healthy adults.

Greater attention must be paid to the social aspects of the disease. Parents and other family members need to have the resources to get the information they so desperately need about their child's diagnosis. Siblings need to know that they are not alone in their own important battles. Patients need to be able to get the best care available, while still getting to play and learn and interact with others around them. Great strides are being made in the right direction, as physicians and other healthcare providers realize the importance of life as a whole, not just life with cancer.

The resources listed in the Appendix are varied. Some provide information about cancer in general or about specific cancer subtypes. Others provide information about social networks for cancer patients and their families. They are not all-inclusive, merely a representation of organizations that attempt to help children and families fighting pediatric cancer.

I hope that this book has provided useful information for those wanting to learn more about the various aspects of pediatric cancer. Maybe some of the "mysteries" of medical care have been explained to families who have become unwillingly immersed in all aspects of the healthcare system. I want this book to be a useful resource for anyone who wants or needs to learn more about the complexities of pediatric cancer.

# Appendix

# RESOURCES FOR CHILDREN, ADOLESCENTS, AND PARENTS DEALING WITH PEDIATRIC CANCER

## GENERAL PEDIATRIC CANCER INFORMATION

American Cancer Society—Children and Cancer: Information and Resources ( http://www.cancer.org/docroot/CRI/CRI_2_6x_Children_and_Cancer.asp) 1-800-ACS-2345
*Links to details about childhood cancer and its treatment and detection. Also discusses some psychosocial issues and support information for children and families dealing with childhood cancer.*

CureSearch—National Childhood Cancer Foundation Children's Oncology Group
http://www.curesearch.org
*Provides information for parents, families, and patients about different types of pediatric and adolescent cancer. Also discusses childhood cancer research, certain types of cancer treatment, and psychosocial issues related to cancer. Fund-raising opportunities for childhood cancer as well.*

National Cancer Institute (NCI)—Childhood Cancers
http://www.cancer.gov/cancertopics/types/childhoodcancers

*Up-to-date information about different types of childhood cancers, their treatment and prevention, and links to clinical research trials for each type of cancer.*

## DISEASE-SPECIFIC INFORMATION

Children's Brain Tumor Foundation
http://cbtf.org
1-866-228-4673
274 Madison Avenue Suite 1004
New York, NY 10016

*Created by parents and physicians for patients with childhood brain tumors. Provides information about the diagnosis, treatment, and after treatment effects of brain tumors. Some publications available for patients and families.*

Children's Neuroblastoma Cancer Foundation
http://www.cncf-childcancer.org
1-866-671-2623
P.O. Box 6635
Bloomingdale, IL 60108

*Information for families of children with neuroblastoma. Foundation that raises money for medical research in the area of neuroblastoma.*

National Marrow Donor Program (NMDP)
http://www.marrow.org
1-800 MARROW2 (1-800-627-7692)
Suite 500
3001 Broadway Street Northeast
Minneapolis, MN 55413-1753

*Information and resources for donors, patients, and physicians about bone marrow/stem cell and cord blood transplants.*

National Wilms' Tumor Study Group
http://www.nwtsg.org
1-800-553-4878/1-206-667-4842
1100 Fairview Ave. N, M2-A876
PO Box 19024
Seattle, WA 98109-1024

*Designed to give information and support for survivors of Wilms' tumor. Supported through Fred Hutchinson Cancer Research Center and the National Cancer Institute (NCI).*

New Approaches to Neuroblastoma Therapy (NANT)
http://www.nant.org
1-323-361-5687
4650 Sunset Boulevard, MS-54
Los Angeles, CA 90027-6016
*Consortium of 13 universities and children's hospitals that specialize in research and treatment programs for neuroblastoma. Funded through the National Cancer Institute (NCI). Has specific clinical trials available for treatment of high-risk neuroblastoma patients.*

Pediatric Brain Tumor Consortium
http://www.pbtc.org
*Cooperative research organization devoted to research and treatment of pediatric brain tumors. Group was formed through the National Cancer Institute (NCI). Specific clinical trials available for certain pediatric brain tumor patients.*

Pediatric Brain Tumor Foundation
http://www.pbtfus.org
1-800-253-6530
302 Ridgefield Court
Asheville, NC 28806
*Information for patients and parents of patients with brain tumors. Survivor and patient stories. Foundation that provides non-governmental funding for childhood brain tumor research.*

Retinoblastoma.com
http://www.retinoblastoma.com
*A parent's guide to understanding retinoblastoma.*

The Childhood Brain Tumor Foundation
http://www.childhoodbraintumor.org
1-301-515-2900/1-877-217-4166
20312 Watkins Meadow Drive
Germantown, MD 20876

*Information regarding pediatric brain tumors, including events, fundraising, research, and patient stories.*

The Leukemia & Lymphoma Society
http://www.leukemia-lymphoma.org
1-800-955-4572
*Specific information about various types of leukemias and lymphomas. Links to support groups, discussion boards, and fund-raising events.*

## LATE EFFECTS OF CANCER THERAPY

Beyond the Cure
https://www.beyondthecure.org
1-314-241-1600
1015 Locust St., Suite 600
St. Louis, MO 63101
*Through the National Children's Cancer Society, provides information about late effects in cancer survivors, specific to diagnosis and treatment.*

Long-Term Follow-Up Guidelines for Survivors of Childhood, Adolescent, and Young Adult Cancer
http://www.survivorshipguidelines.org
*Written guidelines for people who have undergone any type of treatment for childhood cancer. Gives recommendation for follow-up studies, testing, and interventions for treatment-related effects. Provided by the Children's Oncology Group.*

## PEDIATRIC ONCOLOGIST GROUPS

American Society of Pediatric Hematology / Oncology
http://www.aspho.org
1-847-375-4716
*Link for finding a local Pediatric Hematologist/Oncologist and meetings discussing pediatric cancer.*

## PARENT-SPONSORED GROUPS

Candlelighters Childhood Cancer Foundation
http://www.candlelighters.org
1-800-366-CCCF (2223)
P.O. Box 498
Kensington, MD 20895-0498

*Created by parents of children with cancer. Information for patients and parents about childhood cancer. Gives information regarding pediatric cancer advocacy, support, research, and fundraising.*

## AIR TRANSPORT SUPPORT

The Air Care Alliance
http://aircareall.org
1-888-260-9192
1515 East 71st Street, Suite 312
Tulsa, Oklahoma 74136
   *Provides air transportation to patients who qualify under certain circumstances with volunteer pilots and charitable aviation groups.*

Air Charity Network
http://aircharitynetwork.org
1-877-621-7177
   *Provides access to people in need seeking free air transportation to specialized health care facilities at distant destinations due to family, community, or national crisis.*

National Patient Travel Center
http://www.patienttravel.org
1-800-296-1217
   *Facilitates patient access to appropriate charitable medical air transportation resources in the United States. Nation Patient Travel HELPLINE program.*

## PEDIATRIC CANCER ADVOCACY

Hope Street Kids
http://www.hopestreetkids.org
   *Provides facts about childhood cancer, advocacy for cancer patients, and information regarding grants, research, and fundraising.*

National Children's Cancer Society
http://www.nationalchildrenscancersociety.com
1-314-241-1600
1015 Locust St., Suite 600
St. Louis, MO 63101

*Non-profit organization based in St. Louis, looking to improve quality of life for children with cancer and their families. Provides direct financial aid, in-kind assistance, advocacy, support, and education.*

The Children's Cause for Cancer Advocacy
http://www.childrenscause.org
1-301-562-2765
1010 Wayne Avenue, Suite 770
Silver Spring, MD 20910
   *Advocacy organization looking for therapies for childhood cancers and improved quality of life for cancer survivors.*

## HOSPICE CARE AND GRIEF RESOURCES

Children's Hospice International
http://www.chionline.org
1-800-24CHILD
1101 King Street, Suite 360
Alexandria, VA 22314
   *Non-profit organization that promotes hospice support through pediatric care facilities and provides education, training, and technical assistance for those who take care of children with life-threatening conditions.*

The Compassionate Friends
http://www.compassionatefriends.org
1-877-969-0010/1-630-990-0010
PO Box 3696
Oak Brook, IL 60522-3696
   *Information for families dealing with grief following the death of a child.*

## SUPPORT GROUPS AND PATIENT ACTIVITIES

Caring Bridge
http://www.caringbridge.org
1-651-452-7940
CaringBridge
1995 Rahn Cliff Curt, Suite 200
Eagan, MN 55122
   *Free, personalized Web sites for patients and families dealing with critical illnesses, treatment, and recovery. Excellent resource for keeping loved ones up to*

*date about health issues. Includes areas for patient photos, daily journal, and guestbook.*

Children's Oncology Camping International
http://www.coca-intl.org
1-515-491-4999
PO Box 41433
Des Moines, Iowa 50309
   *Information regarding pediatric cancer camps that are available for patients with cancer. Links to local camps for children and adolescents, conferences, and resources about childhood cancer.*

Make-A-Wish Foundation
http://www.wish.org
1-800-722-WISH (9474)
3550 North Central Avenue, Suite 300
Phoenix, Arizona 85012-2127
   *Program that grants "wishes" to children with life-threatening conditions such as cancer. This organization has been granting wishes since 1980, and more than 150,000 children have been helped by this organization.*

Starlight Starbright Children's Foundation
http://www.starlight.org
(310) 479-1212
5757 Wilshire Blvd., Suite M100
Los Angeles, CA 90036
   *Provides a social network for children with chronic illnesses, allowing patients to contact others, such as siblings or other patients. Also offers computer-based information for patients and their families on topics such as chemotherapy and medical tests.*

## FINANCIAL ASSISTANCE ORGANIZATIONS

Kelly Anne Dolan Memorial Fund
http://www.kadmf.org
1-215-643-0763
PO Box 556, 602 S. Bethlehem Pike, Bldg D, 2$^{nd}$ Floor
Ambler, PA 19002
   *Information and resources for uninsured families needing financial assistance to care for seriously ill and physically challenged children.*

The National Children's Cancer Society
http://www.nationalchildrenscancersociety.org

*Provides financial assistance, support services, and education for families dealing with childhood cancer.*

# NOTES

## CHAPTER 2: TYPES OF CANCER, PART I—LEUKEMIA

1. Ries LAG, Smith MA, Gurney JG, Linet M, Tamra T, Young JL, Bunin GR (eds). *Cancer Incidence and Survival among Children and Adolescents: United States SEER Program 1975-1995*, National Cancer Institute, SEER Program. NIH Pub. No. 99-4649. Bethesda, MD, 1999.

2. Ibid.

3. Ibid.

## CHAPTER 3: TYPES OF CANCER, PART II—LYMPHOMA

1. Ries LAG, Smith MA, Gurney JG, Linet M, Tamra T, Young JL, Bunin GR (eds). *Cancer Incidence and Survival among Children and Adolescents: United States SEER Program 1975-1995*, National Cancer Institute, SEER Program. NIH Pub. No. 99-4649. Bethesda, MD, 1999.

2. Ibid.

3. Ibid.

4. Ibid.

5. Ibid.

## CHAPTER 4: TYPES OF CANCER , PART III—BRAIN TUMORS, NEUROBLASTOMA, AND KIDNEY TUMORS

1. Ries LAG, Smith MA, Gurney JG, Linet M, Tamra T, Young JL, Bunin GR (eds). *Cancer Incidence and Survival among Children and Adolescents: United States SEER Program 1975-1995*, National Cancer Institute, SEER Program. NIH Pub. No. 99-4649. Bethesda, MD, 1999.

2. Ibid.
3. Ibid.
4. Ibid.
5. Ibid.
6. Ibid.

## CHAPTER 5: TYPES OF CANCER, PART IV—BONE TUMORS, AND MUSCLE TUMORS

1. Ries LAG, Smith MA, Gurney JG, Linet M, Tamra T, Young JL, Bunin GR (eds). *Cancer Incidence and Survival among Children and Adolescents: United States SEER Program 1975-1995*, National Cancer Institute, SEER Program. NIH Pub. No. 99-4649. Bethesda, MD, 1999.

2. Ibid.

## CHAPTER 6: TYPES OF CANCER, PART V—RARE PEDIATRIC CANCER DIAGNOSES

1. Ries LAG, Smith MA, Gurney JG, Linet M, Tamra T, Young JL, Bunin GR (eds). *Cancer Incidence and Survival among Children and Adolescents: United States SEER Program 1975-1995*, National Cancer Institute, SEER Program. NIH Pub. No. 99-4649. Bethesda, MD, 1999.

2. Ibid.
3. Ibid.
4. Ibid.
5. Ibid.

# INDEX

Abdominal pain: chemotherapy and, 97; hepatocellular carcinoma and, 52; leukemia and, 8, 17; lymphoma and, 19; mucositis and, 120; renal tumors and, 36

Absolute neutrophil count, 117–118

Actinomycin-D, 95

Acupuncture, 89, 134, 136

Acute leukemia, 7–8, 10–16. *See also* Acute lymphoblastic leukemia; Acute myelogenous leukemia

Acute lymphoblastic leukemia (ALL), 10–13, 25, 142; B-cell ALL, 11–13; chemotherapy for, 85, 87, 90, 91, 97; Down syndrome and, 12; epidemiology of, 10; genetics of, 11–12; pre-B ALL, 11–13; signs and symptoms of, 10; survival in, 12; T-cell ALL, 11–13; treatment of, 12–13

Acute myelogenous leukemia (AML) 13–16, 99, 128; Down syndrome and, 15; epidemiology of, 13; genetics of, 15; M3 subtype, 15;

signs and symptoms of, 13; survival in, 15; treatment of, 15–16

Adjuvant therapy, 86

Adolescents and cancer, 66–67

Adriamycin. *See* doxorubicin

Adult oncology, 3–4; radiation therapy and, 101–102

ALCL. *See* Anaplastic large cell lymphoma

Alkylating agents, 15, 93, 95–96, 98

Allogeneic transplant, 110–11, 112

Alpha-fetoprotein (AFP), 52, 58

Alternative therapies, 131–38, 142–43. *See also* Complementary and alternative medicine

Alveolar rhabdomyosarcoma, 45

Alveolar soft part sarcoma, 44, 46

Amputation, 41, 66, 124, 143, 166

Anaplastic astrocytoma, 31

Anaplastic large cell lymphoma, 25

ANC. *See* Absolute neutrophil count

Anemia, 6–7, 16, 36, 90, 95, 120

Angiosarcoma, 46

Anthracyclines, 15, 92–93

## About the Author

**DELLA L. HOWELL, M.D.** is a Pediatric Hematologist/Oncologist in San Antonio, Texas, overseeing the care of patients with cancer and other blood disorders. She earned her medical degree at Virginia Commonwealth University, completed her Internship and Residency in Pediatrics at the San Antonio Military Pediatric Consortium, and completed a Fellowship in Pediatric Hematology/Oncology at Emory University. Herself a cancer patient, she has a special interest in day-to-day aspects of life with cancer, including innovative cancer treatments and psychosocial issues for cancer patients and long-term survival. Howell lives in Texas with her husband of 12 years and her three young children.